Essential Equations for Anaesthesia

Key Clinical Concepts for the FRCA and EDA

Essential Equations for Anaesthesia

Key Clinical Concepts for the FRCA and EDA

Authors

Dr Edward T. Gilbert-Kawai MBChB

Anaesthetic Registrar, Central London School of Anaesthesia, UK

Dr Marc D. Wittenberg MBChB, BSc (Hons), FRCA

Senior Anaesthetic Registrar, Central London School of Anaesthesia, UK

Foreword and contents editor

Dr Wynne Davies MBBCh, DRCOG, DCH, FRCA, FFICM

University College London Hospitals NHS Foundation Trust, UK

Statistical editor

Dr Rebecca Gilbert PhD

School of Social and Community Medicine, University of Bristol, UK

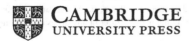

CAMBRIDGE
UNIVERSITY PRESS

CAMBRIDGE
UNIVERSITY PRESS

University Printing House, Cambridge CB2 8BS, United Kingdom

Cambridge University Press is part of the University of Cambridge.

It furthers the University's mission by disseminating knowledge in the pursuit of
education, learning and research at the highest international levels of excellence.

www.cambridge.org
Information on this title: www.cambridge.org/9781107636606

First published 2014

A catalogue record for this publication is available from the British Library

Library of Congress Cataloging-in-Publication Data
Gilbert-Kawai, Edward T.
    Essential equations for anaesthesia : key clinical concepts for the FRCA and EDA / authors,
Dr. Edward T. Gilbert-Kawai, MBChB, Central London School of Anaesthesia, UK, Dr. Marc D. Wittenberg,
MBChB, BSc (Hons), FRCA, Central London School of Anaesthesia, UK ; foreword and contents editor,
Dr. Wynne Davies, MBBCh, DRCOG, DCH, FRCA, FFICM, University College London Hospitals NHS
Foundation Trust, UK, statistical editor, Dr. Rebecca Gilbert, PhD, School of Social and Community
Medicine, University of Bristol, UK.
       pages cm
Includes index.
ISBN 978-1-107-63660-6 (Paperback)
1. Anesthesia–Examinations, questions, etc.   2. Anesthesiology–Examinations, questions, etc.
I. Wittenberg, Marc D.   II. Davies, Wynne (David Wynne Lloyd)   III. Gilbert, Rebecca.   IV. Title.
RD82.3.G55 2014
617.9′6076–dc23   2013045304

ISBN 978-1-107-63660-6 Paperback

....

To those nearest and dearest to me, to Ma for her omniscient advice, and above all to Grace for putting up with me.
Ned Gilbert-Kawai

To my parents for their unwavering love and support, to Eytan and Noa for showing me what life is about, and most of all to my rock, Dalya, without whom none of this would be possible.
Marc Wittenberg

Contents

SECTION 1 – PHYSICS

Part 1a Gases

Part 1b Pressure and flow

Foreword

Sitting examinations is a stressful time; answers are often all too apparent in the coffee room chat following the exit from the examination hall. The way we retrieve and process information has changed. The long evenings spent in the library browsing the *Index Medicus* are fortunately long gone, and have been replaced by much more instant online resources. The information revolution continues, and as wireless technology becomes universal, so access to information will become even more instant.

However, interpretation and emphasis is always going to need guidance. Deriving and remembering equations is a daunting task, particularly when trying to relate them to a clinical context; this book brings together many of the mathematical concepts in anaesthesia into one place. It is an invaluable reference guide to the equations used in anaesthesia today, with a brief explanation of units, and examples of each equation's relevance to clinical practice.

While the authors have attempted to include all equations relevant to post-graduate anaesthetic exams, it is not a panacea for all formulae, but a concise reference text for revision purposes. Succinct and clearly laid out, it enables candidates to build on their academic knowledge, and provides a fresh insight into the clinical applications of the mathematical concepts relevant to anaesthesia.

Doctors Gilbert-Kawai and Wittenberg's *Essential Equations for Anaesthesia* successfully complements other key medical texts as an equation reference guide that will be indispensable to all trainees in anaesthesia, and a refresher for those of us who took the examinations some time ago, before the advent of the information technology revolution.

Dr Wynne Davies MBBCh, DRCOG, DCH, FRCA, FFICM

Preface

One must divide one's time between politics and equations. Equations however are much more important to me, for whilst politics concerns the present, our equations are for eternity.

Albert Einstein (1879–1955)

As practising anaesthetic registrars, we are keenly aware of the challenges and pressures faced by all trainees taking the anaesthetic examinations. Among the seemingly insurmountable mountain of facts and figures that one is expected to know relating to physiology, pharmacology, physics and statistics, knowledge of equations and their derivation, use and application to anaesthetics is an absolute prerequisite.

Unfortunately, while commonly regarded by candidates as a 'nightmare exam question', this is often a favourite with examiners, particularly in the spoken *viva* exams. Easy marks to win if one can demonstrate their knowledge through a straightforward, clinically applied approach, or easy marks to lose if poorly answered. Learned by rote, attempts to derive and link their application to clinical practice can leave a candidate floundering – a huge forfeiture in an exam where every mark counts.

With this in mind, and having had to refer to nearly 20 books and multiple websites while undertaking our own revision, none of them contained a comprehensive list of the multitude of different equations that we were required to know. And thus it was, during a coffee break between theatre lists, that the idea of this book was born: a simple, handy, reference guide to all the equations required for the anaesthetics examination, with concise explanations and examples of their direct relevance to clinical practice.

The book is broadly divided into the four subject areas of physics, physiology, pharmacology and statistics. Each equation is explained, derived where necessary, and a worked or clinically relevant example provided to demonstrate its use. Units and relevant terms are given and, where required, clear, concise diagrams have also been provided to simplify understanding. For general interest, the historical background relating to an equation's nomenclature has also been given wherever possible. We expect readers to use it as a source of reference, and enablement to relate the equations to clinical anaesthesia and intensive care medicine.

Our hope is that a clearer understanding of the topic will significantly diminish the fear around this important aspect of the exam. Indeed, it is also hoped that this book will be of use not only to those preparing for examinations, but also to practising anaesthetists, as many of the equations in this book are directly relevant to clinical practice.

Because thorough preparation for any examination cannot be dependent on one text alone, this book is intended to complement, rather than supplant, other reference works, and is not a replacement for robust knowledge. Nor is there any substitute for hard work. Our intention is that using this book will smooth your passage towards successful completion of the examinations and we wish you good luck: if you are reading this, it means there is light at the end of the tunnel.

EG-K and MW
October 2013

Acknowledgements

We very gratefully acknowledge the guidance and support given to us by Dr Wynne Davies. His role in editing the book's content and continuous encouragement has been invaluable in bringing this book to life.

We also express our deep thanks to Dr Rebecca Gilbert for her advice and editorial role on the statistics section.

Boyle's law

PV = K

Or

$$V \propto \frac{1}{P}$$

(at a constant temperature)

Definition of terms used

P = pressure
V = volume
K = constant

Units

None.

Explanation

Boyle's law (Robert Boyle, 1662) describes one of the characteristics of an ideal gas. It states that if the temperature of the gas is held constant, then pressure and volume are inversely proportional.

An ideal gas is a theoretical gas that obeys the universal gas equation (refer to page 9).

Clinical application/worked example

1. *You are asked to transfer a patient that requires 15 l/minute of oxygen and there is one full E-cylinder of oxygen available. How long will this last?*

Boyle's law can be used to determine the amount of oxygen available from a cylinder (V_2), as follows:

The volume (V_1) of an E-cylinder is 10 l.

The pressure (P_1) inside the cylinder is 13,700 KPa. This is the gauge pressure so atmospheric pressure must be added to make absolute pressure of 13,800 KPa.

The atmospheric pressure (P_2) is 100 KPa.

The temperature is constant in both as long as the gas is allowed to expand slowly.

Boyles law states	$P_1 \times V_1 = \text{constant}$
And thus	$P_2 \times V_2 = \text{constant}$
Therefore	$P_1 \times V_1 = P_2 \times V_2$
So	$V_2 = (P_1 \times V_1)/P_2$
Replacing with values	$V_2 = (13,800 \times 10)/100$
	$V_2 = 1,380 \, l$

Therefore, if a full E-cylinder of oxygen were being used in these conditions at a flow-rate of 15 l/minute, it would last approximately 92 minutes.

Bear in mind that 10 l will be left in the cylinder when it runs out.

Charles' law

$$\frac{V}{T} = K$$

Or

$$V \propto T$$

(at a constant pressure)

Definition of terms used

V = volume
T = temperature
K = constant

Units

None.

Explanation

Charles' law (Jacques Charles, 1780) describes one of the characteristics of an ideal gas. It states that if the pressure of a fixed mass of gas is held constant, then the volume and temperature are proportional.

An ideal gas is a theoretical gas that obeys the universal gas equation (refer to page 9).

Texts differ as to the nomenclature of the second perfect gas law. It was first published by Joseph Louis Gay-Lussac in 1802, although he credited the discovery to unpublished work from 1780s by Jacques Charles.

Clinical application/worked example

1. Spirometry

During pulmonary function testing, a patient will exhale gas at body temperature (37 °C) into a spirometer at room temperature.

Therefore, according to Charles' law, as the temperature drops, the volume of the gas decreases to maintain a constant (K).

For this reason, the terms BTPS and ATPS are used to describe these differing conditions (see box). The volume in the spirometer can be corrected from ATPS to BTPS.

> **BTPS**: Body temperature and pressure, saturated with water vapour
> **ATPS**: Ambient temperature and pressure, saturated with water vapour

2. Heat loss

During anaesthesia, the air around the body is heated by convection. As this happens, according to Charles' law, the volume of the mass of gas increases and therefore rises away from the patient.

Gay-Lussac's law (third gas law)

$$\frac{P}{T} = K$$

Or

$P \propto T$ (at constant volume)

Definition of terms used

P = pressure
T = temperature
K = constant

Units

None.

Explanation

Gay-Lussac's law (Joseph Louis Gay-Lussac, 1802), often described as the third gas law, describes one of the characteristics of an ideal gas. It states that if the volume of a fixed mass of a gas is held constant, then the pressure and temperature are proportional.

An ideal gas is a theoretical gas that obeys the universal gas equation (refer to page 9).

Clinical application/worked example

1. Describe the 'filling ratio' in relation to nitrous oxide cylinders

The filling ratio is calculated as:

$$\frac{\text{weight of the fluid in the cylinder}}{\text{weight of water required to fill the cylinder}}$$

Within a cylinder of gas, according to the third gas law, as the ambient temperature rises, the pressure inside the cylinder will also rise.

This is important in the storage of nitrous oxide with its low Critical Temperature. At room temperature, it is stored in a cylinder as a liquid, with vapour on top. As the temperature rises, the pressure exerted by the vapour, the Saturated Vapour Pressure, also rises. If this exceeds the pressure capacity of the cylinder, then it could explode, as the volume is constant.

For this reason, the filling ratio for nitrous oxide in the UK is 0.75, but in hotter climates is 0.67.

2. Apply the third gas law to the hydrogen thermometer

When a constant volume of hydrogen inside the thermometer is heated, its pressure increases. The measured pressure change is directly proportional to the change in temperature.

Avogadro's equation

$$\frac{V}{n} = K$$

Definition of terms used

V = volume of gas
n = amount of substance of the gas
K = a proportionality constant

Units

None.

Explanation

The equation states 'equal volumes of gases at the same temperature and pressure contain the same number of molecules regardless of their chemical nature and physical properties'.

This number (Avogadro's number) is 6×10^{23} and is described as 1 mole.

1 mole = quantity of a substance containing the same number of particles as there are atoms in 12 g of carbon^{12} = 6×10^{23}.

The mass of gases is different, but the concept of number of molecules, or moles, enables comparison between them.

One mole of any gas at STP occupies 22.4 litres.

STP = Standard Temperature and Pressure
273.15 K = 0 °C
101.325 KPa

Clinical application/worked example

1. Use Avogadro's law to explain how to calibrate a sevoflurane vaporizer.

We know: number of moles = (mass of substance (g)/atomic mass).

The molecular weight of sevoflurane is 200. Therefore, 200 g sevoflurane equals 1 mole and would occupy 22.4 litres at STP.

If a vaporizer contains 20 ml of sevoflurane, this is equivalent to 0.1 mole because the density of sevoflurane is 1 g/ml.

If 1 mole occupies 22.4 litres at STP, then 0.1 mole will occupy 2.24 litres at STP.

If this volume of sevoflurane is fully vaporized in to 224 litres of oxygen, the resulting concentration will be:

2.24/224 = 0.01 = 1%

2. How much liquid agent does a vaporizer use per hour?

Ehrenwerth and Eisenkraft (1993) give the formula:

3 × fresh gas flow (FGF) (l/min) × volume% = ml

Typically, 1 ml of liquid volatile agent yields about 200 ml vapour. This is why tipping is so hazardous, as it discharges liquid agent into the control mechanisms, or distal to the outlet. Minute amounts of liquid agent discharged distal to the vaporizer outlet result in a large bolus of saturated vapour delivered to the patient instantaneously.

Universal gas equation

$$PV = nRT$$

Definition of terms used

P = pressure
V = volume
n = the number of moles of the gas
R = the universal gas constant (8.31 J/K/mol)
T = temperature

Units

None.

Explanation

The universal (or ideal) gas equation describes the behaviour of an ideal gas. It is a combination of Avogadro's law (refer to page 7), Boyle's law (refer to page 1) and Charles' law (refer to page 3).

Clinical application/worked example

1. Calculate the contents of an oxygen cylinder.

The universal gas equation may be used to calculate the contents of an oxygen cylinder.

Referring to the equation, in normal circumstances T is constant at room temperature, V is constant as the cylinder has a fixed volume, and R is by definition a constant. These terms therefore may be practically removed from the equation, and so

$$P \propto n$$

The gauge pressure (P) can thus be used to measure the amount of oxygen remaining in the cylinder (n).

2. Calculate the contents of a nitrous oxide cylinder.

In most circumstances, nitrous oxide is stored below its critical temperature of 36.4 °C. It therefore exists in the cylinder as a vapour in equilibrium with the liquid below it.

To determine how much nitrous oxide remains in a given cylinder, it must be weighed, and the weight of the empty cylinder, known as the tare weight, subtracted. Using Avogadro's law (refer to page 7), the number of moles of nitrous oxide may now be calculated.

Using the universal gas equation as above, the remaining volume can be calculated.

Dalton's law of partial pressures

$$P_{TOTAL} = P_{GAS^A} + P_{GAS^B}$$

Definition of terms used

P_{Total} = total pressure
P_{GAS^A} = partial pressure of gas A
P_{GAS^B} = partial pressure of gas B

Units

Units of pressure.

Explanation

Dalton's law (John Dalton, 1801) states that in a mixture of gases the total pressure is always equal to the sum of the individual partial pressures of the gases present. The pressure of each gas is determined by both the number of molecules present and the total volume occupied, and is independent of the presence of any other gases in a mixture.

Clinical application/worked example

1. Calculate the alveolar partial pressure of oxygen (P_AO_2) given the following conditions:

F_iO_2 = 21%
Body temperature = 37°C
Atmospheric pressure = 100 KPa
P_ACO_2 = 4 KPa

The partial pressure of inspired oxygen (P_iO_2) = F_iO_2 × atmospheric pressure = 0.21 × 100 = 21 KPa.
   However, air in the lungs is saturated with water vapour and mixed with alveolar CO_2.

At 37°C, in normal physiological circumstances, saturated vapour pressure (SVP) of water ≈ 6.3 KPa.

So, using Dalton's law:

$$P_A O_2 = P_i O_2 - (P_A CO_2 + P_A H_2 O)$$
$$= 21 - (4 + 6.3)$$
$$= 10.7 \, KPa$$

2. What is the partial pressure of oxygen at the top of Everest?

Atmospheric pressure (= P_{Total}) at sea level is approximately 101.3 KPa.
Atmospheric pressure (=P_{Total}) at the top of Everest is approximately 33.7 KPa.
The concentration of oxygen is 21%.
Therefore, using Dalton's law, and assuming all other gases being constant:

At sea level, $P_{TOTAL} = P_{O2} + P_{other \, gases}$
$P_{O2} = P_{TOTAL} - P_{other \, gases}$
$P_{O2} = 101.3 - 80.1$
$P_{O2} = 21.2 \, KPa$

On Everest, $P_{TOTAL} = P_{O2} + P_{other \, gases}$
$P_{O2} = P_{TOTAL} - P_{other \, gases}$
$P_{O2} = 33.7 - 26.6$
$P_{O2} = 7.1 \, KPa$

Henry's law

At constant temperature, the mass of a gas that dissolves in a given type and volume of liquid is directly proportional to the partial pressure of that gas in equilibrium with that liquid.

Definition of terms used

Partial pressure = the pressure which the gas would have if it alone occupied the volume of the container.

Units

None.

Explanation

Henry's law (William Henry, 1803) explains that when a liquid is placed into a closed container, with time equilibrium will be reached between the vapour pressure of the gas above the liquid and the liquid itself.

This is equivalent to stating that the solubility of a gas in a liquid is directly proportional to the partial pressure of the gas above the liquid.

Clinical application/worked example

1. Volatile anaesthetic agents

According to Henry's law, the partial pressure of the anaesthetic agent in the blood is proportional to the partial pressure of the volatile in the alveoli. Therefore, if the inspired concentration of volatile agent in the gas mixture is increased, then the concentration in the blood will also increase.

At altitude, this is still the case, as Henry's law also dictates that the only factors that affect the partial pressure of an agent in the blood are:

- the saturated vapour pressure (SVP) of the specific volatile agent;
- its concentration in the alveolus; and
- the ambient temperature.

SVP is not affected by ambient pressure. Standard vaporizer settings do not need to be altered at altitude, except the TEC 6 which is heated and pressurized.

2. Hyperbaric oxygen therapy

Hyperbaric oxygen therapy is used in conditions where it is desirable to increase oxygen delivery, such as decompression sickness, carbon monoxide poisoning, refractory osteomyelitis, or necrotizing wounds.

At sea-level atmospheric pressure breathing room air, the amount of oxygen dissolved in the blood is very small, about 0.3 ml/dl. Under hyperbaric conditions, the partial pressure of oxygen can be significantly increased, and thus according to Henry's law, it means that the concentration of oxygen dissolved in the blood will also increase.

At 3 atmospheres, breathing 100% oxygen, the oxygen concentration in the blood reaches 5.6 ml/dl. This will significantly increase oxygen delivery (refer to page 108), independent of any other factor such as haemoglobin concentration.

Graham's law of diffusion

$$\text{Rate of diffusion} = \frac{1}{\sqrt{MW}}$$

Definition of terms used

MW = molecular weight.

Units

Unit of rate used (mass/time).

Explanation

The rate of diffusion of a gas is inversely proportional to the square root of its molecular weight.

Therefore, the larger the molecule, the slower it diffuses across a membrane.

The equations may relate to diffusion or effusion, depending on the size of the hole in the membrane relative to molecular size. Effusion occurs where individual molecules flow through a hole without collisions with other molecules.

Clinical application/worked example

1. Describe the second gas effect.

This is primarily a concentration effect of rapid uptake of a small molecule thereby concentrating the larger molecule left behind in the alveolus. This facilitates uptake of the second larger molecule.

During induction of anaesthesia, if nitrous oxide is added to the inhaled volatile anaesthetic agent, the alveolar concentration of the volatile anaesthetic agent is increased, thereby accelerating the process.

For example, using nitrous oxide and isoflurane:

MW of N_2O = 44.012 g/mol
MW of isoflurane = 184.5 g/mol

According to Graham's law, nitrous oxide will diffuse across the alveolar membrane in to the blood much more quickly than isoflurane. This in turn increases the concentration of isoflurane in the alveolus, which subsequently increases its partial pressure (refer to Henry's law page 13).

Diffusion hypoxia when discontinuing N_2O is the reverse of this process.

Pressure and force

$$Pressure = \frac{Force}{Area}$$

Or

Force = Pressure × Area

Units

Pressure = Pascal (Pa)
Force = Newton
Area = m^2

Explanation

Force is anything that causes an object to undergo a change in either movement, direction or geometrical construction. It is measured in the SI unit of Newton, as Newton's (Issac Newton, 1687) second law states that 'the net force acting on an object is equal to the rate at which its momentum changes with time'.

Pressure is force per unit area (N/m^2). Because 1 Pascal (Blaise Pascal, 1640s) is approximately equal to the pressure of a piece of paper resting flat on a table, pressures are commonly stated in KPa (1 KPa = 1,000 Pa).

Although the SI unit for pressure is the Pascal, non-SI units are commonly used. For example,

1 KPa = 1 bar = 1 Atm = 14.5 psi = 760 mmHg

Clinical application/worked example

1. Syringes

If we take two syringes of differing size, one 2 ml and the other 20 ml, and fill them with liquid, it is harder to inject from the larger one when applying a constant and equal force. This is because, as the equation states, pressure and area are inversely proportional, thus as the area of the plunger increases, the pressure generated will be less. This equates to more force required to generate the same amount of pressure.

In clinical practice, this is utilized in finding the epidural space because using a wide-bore syringe makes it easier to identify loss of resistance within the low-pressure space. Conversely, unblocking an intravenous catheter is easier with a small syringe as a greater pressure may be achieved.

2. Adjustable pressure limiting (APL) valve

Many breathing circuits contain an APL valve, the aim of which is to adjust and limit the amount of pressure in the circuit during manual or spontaneous ventilation. The valve contains a spring, which can be compressed by turning it, and this in turn exerts a force (F) on diaphragm with an appropriate area (A) within the valve. In order for the valve to open, a certain pressure (P) must be generated, which can be calculated using the equation.

3. Further examples include gauge and absolute pressures

These are described by Boyle's law (refer to page 1).

Hagen–Poiseuille equation (and laminar flow)

$$Q = \frac{\pi P d^4}{128 \eta l}$$

Or

$$Q = \frac{\pi P r^4}{8 \eta l}$$

Definition of terms used

Q = flow
P = pressure drop along the tube
d = diameter of the tube
r = radius of the tube
η = viscosity of the fluid
l = length of the tube
$\pi/128$ = proportionality constant if **diameter** is used in the calculation
$\pi/8$ = proportionality constant if **radius** is used in the calculation

Units

Units can be multiple.

Flow is the mass of a fluid passing a point in unit time.

Units of viscosity are Pascal seconds (Pa·s).

Viscosity is defined as the resistance a fluid offers to the motion of a solid passing through it. It may be dynamic (Pa·s) or kinematic (m^2/s).

Explanation

The Hagen–Poiseuille (Gotthilf Heinrich Ludwig Hagen & Jean Louis Marie Poiseuille, 1840) equation is used to describe the characteristics of laminar flow through a tube. The fluid moves steadily, and all the particles follow the same line of flow in parallel layers (streamlines).

It demonstrates that as the pressure differential along the tube increases, so does flow, and also that flow is inversely proportional to viscosity and length.

Perhaps most importantly, the equation states that as the diameter or radius of the tube increases, flow increases by the fourth power. This means that if the radius doubles, then flow will increase by 16 times.

The equation only applies to Newtonian fluids, which include water but not blood. Those are where the viscosity of the fluid is constant regardless of the accelerating forces in the streamlines.

Clinical application/worked example

1. Intravenous cannulas

The larger the cannula, the faster the flow, increasing by the fourth power of the radius. This explains why wider-bore cannulas, of the same length, have much higher flow rates.

For example, the stated flow rate through a blue 22G cannula is 31 ml/min and 1,000 ml crystalloid will take 32 minutes to infuse. Contrast this with an orange 14G cannula, which has a stated flow rate of 270 ml/min and through which 1,000 ml of crystalloid will take about 3.5 minutes to infuse.

Also, a longer cannula of the same gauge, for example that in a central venous catheter, will have slower flow because length (l) and flow (Q) are inversely related. For this reason, standard multi-lumen central venous catheters are inappropriate for rapid infusion of fluids or blood products in the emergency situation.

2. Endotracheal tubes and anaesthetic breathing circuits

As long as gas flow through an endotracheal tube is laminar, the larger the tube, the less resistance there is to flow. This may be relevant when patients are breathing spontaneously via an endotracheal tube because a narrower tube will increase the work of breathing.

Anaesthetic breathing circuits are designed to maintain laminar flow as much as possible, and reduce the work of breathing for spontaneously ventilating patients. Connections are kept straight, if possible, as acute angles can cause turbulent flow. Also, unnecessarily long circuits will reduce flow. (Refer to page 21.)

3. Anaesthetic machine flowmeters

Flowmeters consist of a vertical tapered glass tube containing a ball or bobbin which floats on the stream of gas. At low flow rates, the tube is narrower and under these circumstances, flow is laminar and respects the Hagen–Poiseuille equation.

Reynold's number (and turbulent flow)

$$Re = \frac{\rho v d}{\eta}$$

Definition of terms used

Re = Reynold's number
ρ = density of the fluid
v = velocity of the fluid
d = diameter of the tube
η = viscosity of the fluid

Units

Because the units of the equation cancel each other out, Reynold's number is dimensionless, i.e. it has no units.
Units of density are usually kg/m^3.

Explanation

Reynold's number (Osborne Reynolds, 1883) describes the factors that determine the critical velocity when flow becomes turbulent rather than laminar. In this instance, the Hagen–Poiseuille equation (refer to page 19) no longer applies.

Turbulent flow refers to a situation in which a fluid moves in a disorganized fashion and begins to swirl, forming eddy currents. As flow is unpredictable, there is no single equation that defines the rate of turbulent flow.

(a) Laminar flow

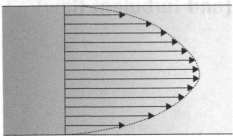

(b) Turbulent flow

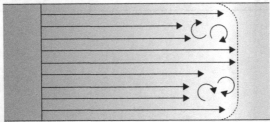

This equation tells us that turbulent flow occurs when fluids flow at high velocity, through large diameter tubes and when fluids are relatively dense.

Density is much more important than viscosity when it comes to turbulent flow. It is defined as the mass of substance occupying a unit volume, as opposed to viscosity which is a measure of its resistance to gradual deformation by shear or tensile stress.

Measurements have shown that when:

- Reynold's number < 2,000, there is likely to be laminar flow;
- Reynold's number 2,000–4,000, there is likely to be transitional flow (laminar and turbulent); and
- Reynold's number > 4000, there is likely to be turbulent flow.

Clinical application/worked example

1. Why is helium used in the management of upper airway obstruction and croup?

In large airways such as the larynx, trachea and large bronchi, flow is generally turbulent because of their large diameter.

Reynold's number dictates that flow in this situation is, among other things, dependent on the density of the gas. In these situations, Heliox (a mixture of 21% oxygen and 79% helium) can be used as it has a significantly lower density than air (0.5 g/l vs. 1.25 g/l at STP). The lower density decreases the Reynold's number, such that there is a higher tendency for flow in the airways to become laminar, thereby decreasing the work of breathing.

In the smaller airways, flow is more likely to be laminar and so Heliox is likely to have a limited effect because laminar flow does not depend on the density of the fluid.

However, caution should be taken using Heliox, as the patient could still be rendered hypoxic due to the low oxygen concentration.

This concept also explains why helium-filled balloons rise, and why inhaling helium will cause your voice to become high-pitched because the flow of gas through the vocal cords is significantly greater!

2. Why do patients with carotid plaques have bruits?

Blood flow through vessels is usually laminar. However, when there is a disruption of flow such as a sharp bend or narrowing, then eddies and currents will form causing turbulent flow.

In the case of carotid atheromas, as blood flows past the plaque, it becomes turbulent and it is this which is audible with a stethoscope as a bruit.

3. Anaesthetic machine flowmeters

Flowmeters consist of a vertical tapered glass tube containing a ball or bobbin which floats on the stream of gas. At higher flow rates, the bobbin moves up the flowmeter until it acts like an orifice and flow becomes turbulent. In this situation the density of the gas affects flow, and hence calibration is gas- or agent-specific.

Flow in this situation becomes proportional to the square root of the pressure and so the graduations on the flowmeter are not uniform.

Laplace's law and tension

$$T = \frac{P \times R}{2t}$$

Or simplified

For a cylinder: $P = \dfrac{T}{R}$

For a sphere with one liquid surface: $P = \dfrac{2T}{R}$

For a bubble with two liquid surfaces: $P = \dfrac{4T}{R}$

Definition of terms used

P = pressure gradient
T = tension
t = wall thickness
R = radius

Units

None.

Explanation

Laplace's (Pierre-Simon Laplace, 1806) law is a principle of physics stating that the tension on the wall of a sphere is the product of the pressure times the radius of the chamber and the tension is inversely related to the thickness of the wall.

The law explains that as the radius of a tube or sphere increases, the pressure gradient across the wall decreases. It also states that as the surface tension increases, the pressure gradient across the wall also increases.

Clinical application/worked example

1. Aortic aneurysms (tubes)

Laplace's cylinder law explains that as the radius of the aorta increases, the tension across its wall also increases so as to maintain the pressure gradient. As tension increases, the risk of rupture increases, and thus abdominal aneurysms larger than 5 cm require urgent repair.

2. Alveolar surfactant (spheres)

The amount of pressure required to inflate an alveolus is dictated by its surface tension and radius. Surfactant, which is normally secreted by type II alveolar epithelial cells, acts to reduce the surface tension.

Therefore, by Laplace's sphere law, the pressure required to inflate the alveolus is significantly reduced. This results in an increase in lung compliance and reduces the tendency for alveoli with smaller radii to collapse in favour of larger ones. Surfactant also reduces fluid leak from pulmonary capillaries across the alveolar wall because the reduced surface tension reduces the hydrostatic pressure gradient across the wall.

Laplace's law also explains why a baby's first breath requires a very large negative intrathoracic pressure and why premature babies with reduced surfactant are prone to lung disease.

Bernoulli equation and Venturi effect

$$P + \frac{1}{2}\rho v^2 + \rho g h = constant$$

Definition of terms used

P = pressure
ρ = density
v = velocity of fluid
g = acceleration due to gravity
h = height of the tube

Units

Units of each term are varied, but as they refer to a constant they are not important in describing the equation.

Explanation

For an ideal fluid, i.e. (i) non-compressible, (ii) non-viscous and (iii) flowing in a laminar fashion, the sum of the pressure (p), kinetic ($\frac{1}{2}\rho v^2$) and potential ($\rho g h$) energies per unit volume remains constant at all points.

Put simply, in order to abide by the law of conservation of energy, the total energy within a fluid system must always remain constant. Therefore, if the kinetic energy (velocity) of the fluid increases, then the potential energy (pressure) will simultaneously fall.

In practical terms, the acceleration of fluid due to gravity can be discounted as we are referring to a horizontal tube. Furthermore, the density of fluid will remain the same, as will the height of the tube.

Thus, the equation can be simplified to:

$$P + \frac{1}{2}\rho v^2 = constant$$

Therefore, the Bernoulli principle (Daniel Bernoulli, 1738) states that if there is an increase in the velocity of an ideal fluid, then there will be a proportional decrease in its pressure.

Clinical application/worked example

1. Venturi effect and Venturi masks

The Venturi effect (Giovanni Battista Venturi, 1797) is a direct consequence of the Bernoulli principle. It describes the effect by which a constriction to fluid flow through a tube causes the velocity of the fluid to increase and therefore the pressure to decrease.

This principle is used in the design of Venturi masks. These are used as fixed performance oxygen delivery devices or as nebulizer devices.

The pressure drop that is caused by the narrow tube allows for entrainment of room air, or liquids as in nebulizer devices. This occurs as a fixed ratio; hence, the concentration of oxygen delivered is independent of the flow rate but dependent on the entrainment ratio, i.e. the relative size of the entrainment hole.

Entrainment ratio = entrained flow/driving flow

The nozzle can have a fixed or variable aperture that is used to set the concentration of oxygen that is delivered.

Ohm's law, voltage, current and resistance

V = IR

Definition of terms used

V = voltage (= electric potential difference = electromotive force)
I = current
R = resistance or impedance

Units

Unit of voltage = Volts (V)
Unit of current = Amperes (A)
Unit of resistance = Ohms (Ω)

Explanation

Ohm's law (Georg Ohm, 1827) is fundamental to understanding the relationship between voltage, current and resistance. It states that for good conductors, the electric current is directly proportional to the potential difference applied, provided that temperature and other physical factors remain constant. The equation can be used to calculate an unknown variable when the other two are known. It is important to remember that when R is calculated for direct current (DC) it represents resistance; however, when alternating current (AC) is used, R represents impedance. Impedance refers to the opposition of flow affected by both magnitude and phase, unlike resistance which has only magnitude.

When a constant potential difference of 1 V applied between two points of a conductor produces a current of 1 A, a resistance of 1 Ω is said to exist between the points. Within a circuit, resistors can either exist in series or in parallel. A series current is one where the resistors are arranged in a chain so that the current has only one path to take. A parallel circuit is one where the resistors are arranged with their heads connected together and their tails connected together. The voltage across each resistor is the same.

In order to calculate the total resistance within a circuit, the equations are as follows:

Series: $R_T = R_1 + R_2 + R_3 + \ldots$

Parallel: $1/R_T = 1/R_1 + 1/R_2 + 1/R_3 + \ldots$

where
R_T = total resistance
R_n = each resistor in turn up to the total number.

Current describes moving charge, or flow of electrons, and Ohm's law can be thought of as analogous to water flow from a large container through a pipe out of the side of the container that has a constriction within it: V is the height of the water above where the pipe exits the container, I is the speed of the water out of the pipe and R represents the constriction within the pipe. It is easy to see how, if the height of the water increases, then current will increase; and if the constriction in the pipe increases, then the current will decrease.

Therefore, I is proportional to V, and inversely proportional to R.

Clinical application/worked example

1. How does Ohm's law apply to blood pressure?

Ohm's law can easily be applied to the physiological equation BP = CO × SVR, as blood pressure (BP) is equivalent to V, cardiac output (CO) is equivalent to I, and systemic vascular resistance (SVR) is equivalent to R.

It is therefore easy to conceptualize how in a patient with severe sepsis and vasodilatation (decreased R), the cardiac output needs to increase to maintain the blood pressure.

2. How does Ohm's law apply to the Wheatstone bridge?

The Wheatstone bridge is most commonly found in the transducer of an intra-arterial blood pressure monitoring system. The transducer converts one form of energy into another; in this case, change in pressure is measured as a change of resistance within the bridge. It consists of a ring of 4 resistances (R_{1-4}) supplied by a DC voltage across diagonally opposite corners of the ring (A and C).

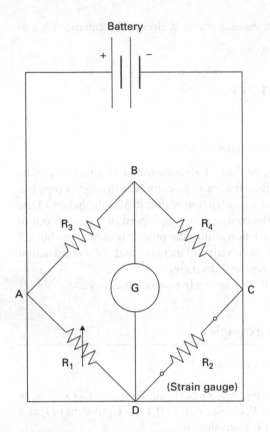

When there is a change of pressure, there is a proportional change in the transducer's resistance (R), which causes a current (I) to flow through the meter. A variable resistor (R_1) changes in order to 'balance the bridge' and it is the magnitude of this change which can be calculated to reflect the pressure change such that:

$$\frac{R_1}{R_3} = \frac{R_2}{R_4}$$

Because R and I are known, Ohm's law can be used to calculate the pressure change, V.

Capacitance and capacitors

$$F = \frac{C}{V}$$

Or

$$E = \frac{1}{2}CV^2$$

Definition of terms used

F = farad (unit of capacitance)
C = coulomb (unit of charge)
V = volt (unit of potential difference of voltage)
E = energy stored by a capacitor

Units

As above.

Explanation

A capacitor is a device that stores electrical charge, and capacitance describes the ability of an object to store that charge (refer to page 39). It is measured in farads (F). The first equation describes the fact that a capacitor with a capacitance of one farad will store one coulomb of charge when one volt is applied across it. The energy then stored by the capacitor can be calculated by the second equation.

Capacitors are fundamental to electrical circuits. They generally consist of two metal plates separated by a non-conducting substance. A simple example would be two pieces of aluminium foil separated by a piece of paper. The plates have a potential difference between them, but cannot conduct direct current (DC) due to the non-conductor. However, capacitors conduct alternating current (AC) well because the plates charge and discharge as the flow of current changes.

Clinical application/worked example

1. Where does capacitance exist in the operating theatre?

Capacitance can exist between everyday objects that act as two metal plates. This includes ECG leads, the patient, the operating table and theatre lights. Air is the non-conducting substance, otherwise known as the dielectric. When two objects act as a capacitor, this is called capacitative coupling, and can result in electrostatic interference.

2. How is a capacitor applied in a defibrillator?

The most important component of a defibrillator is a capacitor. This is because it stores a large amount of charge and then discharges it very quickly to the myocardium. This discharge is an exponential decay and is too quick for complete defibrillation. For successful defibrillation, the current delivered must be maintained for several milliseconds using an inductor (refer to page 33).

Inductance and inductors

$$H = \frac{Wb}{A}$$

Definition of terms used

H = Henry (unit of inductance)
Wb = Weber (unit of magnetic field strength)
A = Ampere (unit of current)

Units

As above.

Explanation

An inductor is an electrical device that opposes changes in current flow through a wire, by means of the generation of an electromotive force (EMF). EMF is analogous to voltage. Inductance arises in circuits with alternating current (AC): as the current continuously reverses, the associated magnetic field in the coiled wire waxes and wanes. In turn, this fluctuating magnetic field induces a current in the coiled wire in the opposite direction to the original current.

The equation describes the fact that one Henry of inductance is generated when one Ampere of current flows through a coil and produces a magnetic field strength of one Weber.

Clinical application/worked example

1. Where are inductors applied in clinical practice?

An inductance coil is present in a defibrillator circuit to prolong the defibrillation phase of discharge of the capacitor, which has a fast exponential decay. For successful defibrillation, the current delivered must be maintained for several milliseconds. However, the current and charge delivered by a discharging capacitor decays rapidly and exponentially. Inductors are therefore used to prolong the duration of current flow.

(a) Unmodified without inductor

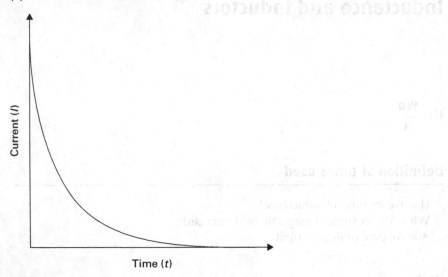

Exponential decay of current over time.

(b) Modified with an inductor

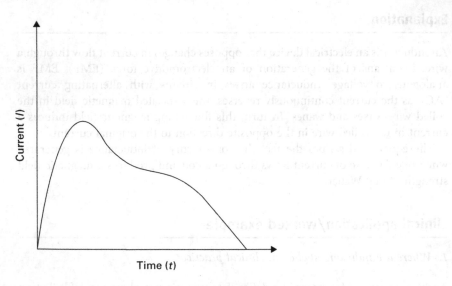

Waveform prolonged after passage through inductor.

Work and power

Work done: $W = F \times D$

Definition of terms used

W = work done
F = force
D = distance

Units

Work = joule (J) = Nm.

Explanation

Work refers to the process by which a force acts on a body to move it in the direction of the force. Energy is thereby expended. The unit, joule, refers to the fact that it measure the amount of work done when a force of 1 newton (N) moves its point of application 1 metre (m) in the direction of that force.

Power refers to the rate of work done, and is defined as the amount of energy, in joules, consumed per unit time. Watts, named after James Watt (1736–1819), is the unit of power. 1 Watt equals 1 Joule per second.

When referring to electrical power, the equation is as follows:

$P = I \times V$

where P = power, I = current and V = potential difference (voltage).

Clinical application/worked example

1. *Discuss the calculation of the work done by the movement of a constant-pressure generator ventilator.*

A ventilator of this nature generates a volume of gas by compressing bellows. The force (F) needed to do so, multiplied by the distance (D) moved by the bellows can be used to calculate the work done using the equation.

The volume of gas (V) delivered is also a product of the distance moved (D) and the area (A) of the bellows. As we know that force, F, is a product of pressure (P) and area (A), these concepts can be combined to deduce that the work done (W) by the ventilator is also a product of the volume of gas moved, and the pressure required, as follows:

$$W = F \times D$$
and $\quad F = P \times A$
and $\quad V = D \times A$
So $\quad D = V/A$

Therefore $\quad$ **W = PA × V/A = PV**

2. Discuss the concepts of power in relation to the heart.

The notion of electrical power can also be applied to the heart in that the power of the heart is a product of the pressure (or potential) difference and the fluid flow (or current).

The pressure difference in the left side is analogous to difference between the mean arterial pressure and pulmonary venous pressure (which is normally 0), and the current can be compared to the cardiac output. Similarly, for the right side of the heart, the pressure difference would equate to mean pulmonary artery pressure minus the right atrial pressure.

Therefore, the power of the heart may be calculated as pressure difference × cardiac output.

Transformers

$$V2 = V1 \times \left(\frac{n1}{n2}\right)$$

Definition of terms used

$V1$: primary voltage
$V2$: secondary voltage
$n1$: number of coils of wire (primary)
$n2$: number of coils of wire (secondary)

Units

Voltage.

Explanation

A transformer is a static electrical device that transfers electrical energy from one circuit to another by inductive coupling. Transformers are used to raise or lower the voltage in a circuit depending on the requirements. An example is the National Grid, where energy is transferred around the country by voltage rather than current in order to reduce heat losses.

In its simplest form, a transformer consists of two lengths of insulated wire, each wound (or coiled up) around an iron core. These coils tend to differ in terms of the number of windings each has. An alternating current in the primary winding creates a varying magnetic flux in the primary transformer's core, subsequently producing a magnetic flux and alternating current in the secondary core and coil, respectively.

In an ideal transformer, i.e. a perfectly coupled one in which there is no loss of energy, the voltage induced in the secondary coil may be calculated from the above formula.

Importantly, the ratio of the electrical current strength, or amperage, in the two coils is inversely proportionate to the ratio of the voltages, and thus the electrical power (voltage multiplied by amperage) is the same in both coils.

Clinical application/worked example

1. Describe the concept of a step-up or step-down transformer.

A transformer consists of two metal cores (termed primary and secondary), each with an insulated wire coiled around it. The ratio of the number of turns in the primary coil to the number of turns in the secondary coil, known as the 'turns ratio', determines the ratio of the voltages in the two coils. For example, in a 'step-up' transformer there may be one turn in the primary coil, and 20 turns in the secondary coil, such that the voltage in the secondary coil will be 20 times that in the primary. Alternatively a 'step-down' transformer will have more turns of wire around the primary core as compared to the secondary core. The voltage induced in one coil may be calculated if the number of coils in each core is known, as well as the initial voltage.

2. Describe the concept of an isolation transformer.

In many pieces of electrical equipment an isolation transformer is used to transfer electrical power from a source of alternating current (AC) power to a piece of equipment or device. This isolates the powered device from the power source. Isolation transformers provide galvanic isolation and are used to protect against electric shock, to suppress electrical noise in sensitive devices, or to transfer power between two circuits which must not be connected. Isolation transformers block transmission of the DC component in signals from one circuit to the other, but allow AC components in signals to pass.

Electrical charge

$Q = I \times T$

Or

$Q = C \times V$

Definition of terms used

Q = charge
I = current
T = time (seconds)
C = capacitance
V = potential difference or voltage

Units

Coulomb.

Explanation

Charge is a fundamental property of matter whereby elementary particles, occurring in discrete natural units, which can neither be created nor destroyed, carry charge that can either be positive or negative. It is measured in Coulombs (Charles-Augustin de Coulomb, 1784) such that one Coulomb describes the net amount of electrical charge that flows through a conductor in a circuit during each second when the current has a value of one ampere (6.24×10^{18} electrons). Like charges repel each other and tend to move from an area of high charge density, or potential, to those of lower potential. The flow of charge is known as electrical current and can be calculated using the first equation by measuring the amount of current that flows multiplied by unit time.

Charge is also a product of capacitance and voltage (refer to page 31). A capacitor stores charge and has a potential difference across its plates.

Clinical application/worked example

1. *List two methods in which electrical charge is used therapeutically or diagnostically.*

(i) Defibrillators: direct current (DC) is applied to a capacitor so that charge builds up on the capacitor plates. As the charge on the plates increases, a potential difference is created.

(ii) Electrical nerve stimulator: stimulators are used to locate peripheral nerves in order to administer regional anaesthesia, or to assess residual neuromuscular blockade. In each case, a certain current is applied for a defined amount of time, thereby allowing calculation of the charge delivered.

Doppler equation and effect

$$v = \frac{cf_d}{2f_T \cos \theta}$$

Definition of terms used

v = flow velocity
c = the speed of sound in tissues
f_d = Doppler frequency shift that is received
$\cos \theta$ = cosine of the angle between the sound beam and moving fluid (45°)
f_T = frequency of the transmitted ultrasound from the transducer (Hz)

Units

m/s.

Explanation

The Doppler equation, although not necessary to memorize, is fundamental to understanding the Doppler effect. When first described by Christian Doppler in 1842, it related to the phenomenon whereby there is a change in frequency for an observer moving relative to the source of a wave.

For example, if a person is standing still and an ambulance approaches, the pitch of the siren changes as the vehicle approaches, passes and moves away.

Clinical application/worked example

1. How is the Doppler effect used to calculate cardiac output?

The Doppler effect is used in the measurement of the velocity of blood cells using the oesophageal Doppler probe (ODP). The cardiac output and other variables are then calculated.

The ultrasound probe contains a transmitter, which transmits ultrasonic waves at frequency f_T, and a receiving transducer, that detects the frequency of the reflected ultrasound waves, f_d.

If red blood cells are moving towards or away from the transducer (like the ambulance siren), then there is Doppler shift. The magnitude of this shift is directly proportional to the velocity (v) of the blood cells.

Note that the cosine of 90° = 0. Therefore, if the probe is perpendicular to the flow of blood, then there will be no Doppler shift. Therefore, the transducer of the ODP is positioned at 45° to the flow of blood in order to assess its velocity. Ideally, a Doppler shift should be parallel to the object being measured for velocity for maximum accuracy; however, the 45° probe on the ODP is a compromise.

Beer–Lambert law

$A = \varepsilon d c$

Definition of terms used

A = absorbance
ε = molar extinction coefficient
d = path length in cm
c = molar concentration

Units

Variable.

Explanation

This is a combination of two laws that combine to form a mathematical means of expressing how light is absorbed by matter.

(1) Beer's law states that: *the intensity of transmitted light decreases exponentially as concentration of the substance increases.*

(2) Lambert's law states that: *the intensity of transmitted light decreases exponentially as the distance travelled through the substance increases.*

Combining the two laws means that the transmission of light through a substance (the inverse of absorbance) is inversely proportional to its molar concentration and thickness.

Clinical application/worked example

1. Give an example of how this law is relevant to anaesthesia?

The Beer–Lambert law is relevant to pulse oximetry – a monitoring technique that works on the basis of spectrophotometry. The pulse oximeter probe, usually placed on a digit, emits light at different wavelengths. The blood absorbs a certain proportion of light, which is dependent on the relative concentrations of deoxy-haemoglobin and oxyhaemoglobin present. A photodetector placed at a constant path length away on the opposite side of the probe (and thus digit) senses the amount of light that has been absorbed and processes this electronically to give oxygen saturation and pulse waveform, or plethysmograph.

The original wavelengths of 640 nm and 990 nm were chosen at the time of invention, not because of scientific reasoning, but because these diodes were commercially available!

Relative humidity

$$\varnothing = \left(\frac{e_\omega}{e *\omega} \right) \times 100$$

Definition of terms used

$\varnothing$ = relative humidity
e_ω = partial pressure of water vapour = absolute vapour pressure
$e * \omega$ = saturated vapour pressure of water at a given temperature

Units

Percentage.

Explanation

Humidity, the mass of water vapour in the air, may be expressed in absolute, relative or specific terms. Absolute humidity is the mass of water vapour per unit volume of air. Specific humidity is the ratio of water vapour to dry air in a set volume. Relative humidity is defined as the ratio of the partial pressure of water vapour in the air at a given time (absolute vapour pressure) to the saturated vapour pressure of water at the present temperature.

Clinical application/worked example

1. How is humidity important in the theatre setting?

Controlled humidity levels in operating theatres provide a comfortable working environment, and minimize patient heat loss and the accumulation of static charges. Relative humidity is kept at 40–60%. Too humid and it becomes uncomfortable; too dry and there is a risk of static electricity and spark generation.

Natural frequency

$$NF \alpha \frac{D}{\sqrt{LCd}}$$

Definition of terms used

NF = natural frequency
D = catheter diameter
L = tube length
C = system compliance
d = fluid density

Units

Hertz (Hz).

Explanation

Every material has a frequency at which it freely oscillates, known as the natural frequency. If a force with a similar frequency to the natural frequency is applied to the system, it will begin to oscillate at its maximum amplitude. This is known as resonance.

Clinical application/worked example

1. *Discuss the application of natural frequency to invasive arterial blood pressure (IABP) monitoring.*

The system set-up for IABP monitoring consists of fluid-filled tubing, which is attached to a bag of pressurized fluid at one end, and an intra-arterial catheter at the other end. This tubing has a natural frequency at which it oscillates.

The arterial waveform is transmitted from the cannula in the artery to the pressure transduced by means of a waveform which is made up of a number of component sine waves. Should the natural frequency of the IABP system lie close to the frequency of any of the sine waves within the arterial waveform, then the system will resonate, causing a distortion of the measurement. Therefore, to avoid resonance at the high heart rates, the frequency response of the monitoring system should exceed 30 Hz.

As can be seen by the equation, the natural frequency of the system is increased by:

- increasing the diameter of the tubing;
- decreasing the tube length;
- reducing the compliance of the tubing; and
- reducing the density of the fluid within the tubing.

Ideally, therefore, arterial cannulae should be short, stiff and wide-bore, but not so wide that they cause distal arterial occlusion. Similarly, the tubing that connects the arterial cannula to the transducer should also be short, stiff and wide-bore; however, for convenience, this is often quite long, although fairly stiff and non-compliant.

Wave equation and ultrasound

$$v = f \times \lambda$$

Definition of terms used

v = velocity
λ = wavelength
f = frequency

Units

m/s.

Explanation

For a sinusoidal wave, the mathematical relationship between the speed (v) of a wave and its wavelength (λ) and frequency (f) is derived by the equation above. Wavelength and frequency can thus be calculated by rearranging the equation. Assuming the sinusoidal wave is propagated at a constant velocity, wavelength is inversely proportional to frequency, such that waves with lower frequencies have longer wavelengths and vice versa.

Clinical application/worked example

1. *Why are frequency and wavelength important for generating clear ultrasound pictures?*

Medical ultrasound uses sound waves with a frequency outside the audible limit of normal human hearing. These are typically above 20,000 Hz, but may rise to 50 MHz.

While ultrasound cannot detect objects that are smaller than its wavelength (and therefore higher frequencies of ultrasound produce better resolution), at a given velocity the choice of frequency is a trade-off between imaging depth and the quality of the image, as higher frequencies are more readily absorbed and therefore do not penetrate as deep into the tissue. As $v = f \lambda$ and $v \approx 1{,}540$ m/s (approximately in human tissue), a probe frequency of 1–15 MHz is required to visualize objects of 1 mm diameter. High frequencies are rapidly attenuated, so there is a trade-off between axial resolution and depth penetration. It is therefore important to select a probe of appropriate frequency for the size and depth of the target.

The smaller the wavelength (and therefore higher the frequency), the higher the resolution, but lesser penetration. Therefore, higher-frequency probes (5–10 MHz) provide better resolution but can be applied only for superficial structures and in children. Lower-frequency probes (2–5 MHz) provide better penetration, albeit lower resolution, and can be used to image deeper structures.

Bioavailability

$$F = \frac{AUC_{po} \times Dose_{iv}}{AUC_{iv} \times Dose_{po}}$$

Definition of terms used

F = fraction absorbed
AUC_{po} = area under the curve – oral route
AUC_{iv} = area under the curve – intravenous route
$Dose_{iv}$ = dose administered – intravenous route
$Dose_{po}$ = dose administered – oral route

Units

Fraction (f) or percent (F).

Explanation

Bioavailability describes the proportion of the administered dose of a drug that reaches the systemic circulation. As, by definition, drugs given intravenously (iv) have a bioavailability of 100%, the iv route is taken as the reference standard to which other routes of administration are compared.

Given that the total amount of drug reaching the systemic circulation is directly proportional to the area under a concentration–time curve (AUC), the bioavailability (F) is determined by comparing respective AUCs. The AUC ratio is corrected for any differences in dose (D) administered, and providing there is no change in drug elimination between administrations, an accurate estimate is obtained.

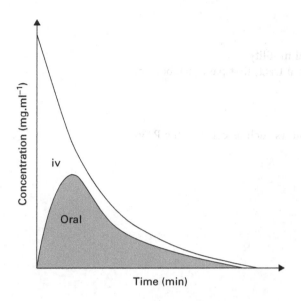

Clinical application/worked example

1. Given the following, calculate the bioavailability of the oral dose of this antibiotic.

$Dose_{po} = 10\,mg$

$Dose_{iv} = 10\,mg$

$AUC_{po} = 4.5\,mg/ml/h$

$AUC_{iv} = 11.2\,mg/ml/h$

$F = (4.5 \times 10)/(11.2 \times 10)$

$F = 0.4$ or 40%

2. What factors affect bioavailability?

Properties of the drug:
- particle size,
- structure,
- solubility,
- pKa,
- hydrophobicity.

Physiological factors:
- gastric pH,
- gastric emptying intestinal motility,
- perfusion of gastrointestinal tract, first pass metabolism.

Pathological factors:
- cardiac and liver disease,
- enzyme inducers or inhibitors such as cytochrome P450,
- vomiting,
- diarrhoea.

Volume of distribution

$$V_d = \frac{X}{C_0}$$

Definition of terms used

V_d = volume of distribution
X = amount of drug in the body (mg)
C_0 = plasma concentration at time zero (mg/l)

Units

Litres.

Explanation

The volume of distribution (V_d) describes the apparent volume into which a drug disperses in order to produce the observed plasma concentration (C_0). In a one-compartment model, Vd is the proportionality constant that relates the amount of drug in the body to plasma concentration at time zero.

V_d is a theoretical volume that has no direct physiological meaning, and in many cases it can be much larger than total body water. It does not correspond to any particular physiological volumes. It is more a reflection of how a drug distributes within the body in relation to its physicochemical properties such as solubility, charge and molecular weight.

Clinical application/worked example

1. *Give examples of volumes of distribution, and describe what affects this?*

Propofol has a very large volume of distribution (up to 60 l/kg). This means that the drug is more dilute than if solely distributed in the plasma alone, and thus it must also be distributed within the tissues. As propofol is extremely lipid-soluble (non-polar) a large proportion is taken up into fatty tissue. Drugs with high V_d also include those that have low rates of ionization, or low plasma-binding capabilities.

Pancuronium, a non-depolarizing muscle relaxant, has a relatively small V_d (260 ml/kg), as does **warfarin** (140 ml/kg). Pancuronium is a highly charged molecule and warfarin has a high degree of plasma protein binding, thus both are not widely distributed.

2. *Calculate the* V_d *for the following theoretical anaesthetic drug given to a patient weighing 60 kg.*

Dose of drug given = 1,000 µg

Plasma concentration = 2 µg/l

$$V_d = \frac{X}{C_0}$$

= 1,000/2 = 500 litres

= 8.33 l/kg

It is likely from this that the drug is highly lipid-soluble as it has a very high V_d.

Clearance

$$Cl = k \times V_d$$

Or

$$Cl = \frac{V_d}{\tau}$$

Definition of terms used

Cl = clearance
k = rate constant (for elimination)
V_d = volume of distribution
τ = time constant

Units

ml/min.

Explanation

Clearance describes the volume of plasma completely cleared of a substance per unit time. It is governed by the processes of metabolism and excretion. In a one-compartment model, clearance is related to the first-order elimination rate constant (k), and mathematically it is calculated by the product of the rate constant and volume of distribution (V_d). Clearance is constant in first-order kinetics, but is variable in zero-order kinetics.

In multi-compartment models, we calculate clearance from a concentration time plot, from the equation:

Cl = dose/area under curve

The second equation describes the relationship between clearance and the time constant (τ). As the time constant is expressed as the inverse of rate constant (refer to page 71), clearance can also be expressed as the ratio of volume of distribution (V_d) to the time constant.

In practical terms, for most drugs, clearance is almost synonymous with renal clearance even though other organs are involved in clearance. If a drug is cleared by more than pathway, that clearance can be calculated for each pathway – for example, renal and hepatic – and then added together to calculate the total clearance.

Clinical application/worked example

1. *Calculate the clearance for drug X that demonstrates first-order kinetics, given the V_d = 10 litres, and k = 0.5/min.*

The rate constant describes the proportion of plasma from which the drug is removed per minute, in this case 50%. Clearance is the product of rate constant and volume of distribution. Therefore:

$10 \times 0.5 = 0.5$ l/min

2. *Give examples of drugs that are 100% renally cleared and explain the implications of renal impairment.*

(i)   **Lithium**: this drug has a narrow therapeutic window. Therefore, in renal impairment, estimates of renal function can be useful in determining if low or high concentrations are due to poor compliance or under- or over-dosing.

(ii) **Allopurinol**: estimates of renal function can be used to guide dosing as well as clinical and biochemical measures of effect, such as serum urate concentration.

(iii) **Amoxicillin**: this drug has a wide therapeutic window and therefore dosing is not normally adjusted for short-term use in patients with renal disease. However, estimates of renal clearance can be useful to identify those patients who may need smaller doses or longer dose intervals.

Hepatic clearance

$$CL_H = Q \times ER$$

where

$$ER = \frac{C_a - C_v}{C_a}$$

Definition of terms used

CL_H = hepatic clearance
Q = hepatic blood flow (normal 1–1.5 l/min)
ER = extraction ratio (range 0–1)
C_a = drug concentration in the hepatic artery + portal vein
C_v = drug concentration in the hepatic vein

Units

ml/min.

Explanation

Hepatic clearance (CL_H) quantifies the loss of drug during its passage through the liver. It is the product of hepatic blood flow multiplied by the extraction ratio (ER).

The extraction ratio is a measure of the organ's relative efficiency in eliminating the drug from the systemic circulation during a single pass through the liver. It can be determined by measuring the concentration of drug entering (C_a) and leaving (C_v) the liver as shown by the equation above.

If the concentration leaving an organ is 0, then the drug has been totally removed from the circulation, and consequently the $ER = 1$. Conversely, if the concentration in C_a is the same as that in C_v then the $ER = 0$.

Clinical application/worked example

1. How does the variation in blood flow to the liver affect clearance?

For drugs with a low extraction ratio (< 0.3) such as warfarin, diazepam and theophylline, the venous drug concentration is virtually identical to the arterial concentration and therefore the liver is poorly influenced by blood flow variations.

For drugs with a high extraction ratio (> 0.7) such as lignocaine, verapamil and propranolol, an increase in blood flow will increase the amount of drug presented to the metabolizing enzymes, and so clearance will increase accordingly.

2. Discuss the factors that may alter liver clearance.

Hepatic clearance is influenced by blood flow entering the organ, and the extraction ratio occurring within the organ. Any condition that affects either of these will alter clearance.

Hepatic blood flow:
- congestive cardiac failure,
- hypovolaemia,
- portal vein thrombosis.

Plasma protein binding:
- hypoalbuminaemia,
- displacement by other drugs.

Hepatic enzyme activity:
- drug inhibition or induction,
- liver failure.

3. Discuss the relationship between extraction ratio and bioavailability.

Drugs with a high *ER* will have a reduced bioavailability due to pre-systemic metabolism in the enterohepatic circulation. These include lignocaine, propranolol and morphine. In the case of morphine, this partly explains why the equivalent oral dose of morphine is approximately double that given iv.

Drugs with a low extraction ratio have negligible first-pass effects, and thus can be given orally. These include warfarin, carbamazepine and diazepam.

Concentration and elimination

$$C = C_0 e^{-kt}$$

Definition of terms used

C = concentration
C_0 = concentration at time zero
t = time
k = rate constant
e = Euler's number (base to the natural logarithm = 2.718)

Units

mg/l or µg/ml.

Explanation

Concentration describes the amount of drug in a given volume of plasma. The equation describes how concentration will change with time in a simple one-compartment model.

Concentration is dependent on time (t), and the relationship is defined by a negative exponential function. Drawn, this would resemble a simple wash-out curve, and the steepness of the curve would depend on the rate constant. As the amount of drug eliminated per unit time is decreasing, the rate constant in this instant is known as the 'elimination' rate constant (or rate constant of elimination). In other words, concentration is never static, but is defined at a certain point in time.

In a multi-compartment model, each compartment will have its own wash-out curve and the resultant graph will be the sum of the negative exponentials (refer to page 65).

Clinical application/worked example

1. Describe how concentration is affected by the rate constant.

The rate constant defines the steepness of the wash-out curve. If all else were to remain constant, and the rate constant doubled, the time for plasma concentration to reach a given value would half. Conversely, if the rate constant is halved, then the time to reach a given plasma concentration would double.

2. Give examples of drugs that satisfy the triexponential model.

- Propofol.
- Fentanyl.
- Thiopentone.

Plasma concentration and compartment models

One-compartment: $C = Ae^{-\alpha t}$

Two-compartment model: $C = Ae^{-\alpha t} + Be^{-\beta t}$

Three-compartment model: $C = Ae^{-\alpha t} + Be^{-\beta t} + Ge^{-\gamma t}$

Definition of terms used

C = plasma concentration
e = Euler's number
A = constant A
B = constant B
G = constant G
$-\alpha t$ = rate constant
$-\beta t$ = rate constant
$-\gamma t$ = rate constant

Units

Units of concentration (mmol/l).

Explanation

In single-compartment modelling, the drug is considered to be distributed instantaneously into a unique compartment in the body.

Multi-compartment models are used to explain the distribution within the body of all intravenous anaesthetic drugs. Although the compartments do not correspond to true physiological structures, in each instance, A represents the central compartment (i.e. plasma) into which a drug is added, and from which excretion can occur. The other compartments (B and G) represent peripheral volumes and the sum of all the compartments is the volume of distribution at steady state.

An intravenous anaesthetic drug will move between the compartments down a concentration gradient, and therefore the rate of change will decrease over time. This can be described by a sum of exponentials.

In a two-compartment model, plasma concentration initially declines with a rapid exponential phase (time constant α). This is predominantly due to early distribution from the first compartment into the second. Once this distribution has occurred, plasma concentration falls at a second slower exponential rate (terminal elimination) determined by time constant β.

In a three-compartment model, an additional compartment is added into the equation, and three exponential processes are required. It is tempting to speculate that compartment B corresponds to a vessel-rich group and compartment G corresponds to a fat and vessel-poor group. This may provide some insight, particularly for highly lipophilic drugs such as the IV anaesthetic agents in which a large G may be explained by extensive distribution into fatty tissues.

Using the equations, and having an awareness of the pharmacokinetic models, it is possible to calculate the overall plasma concentration. However, in reality, the distribution of drugs within the body is considerably more complex than is implied by simple compartmental models.

Clinical application/worked example

1. Describe how target-controlled infusions relate to the three-compartment model.

Target-controlled infusion (TCI) pumps incorporate software that models the various body compartments according to the multi-compartmental model. These are typically derived from measuring the blood concentration of a drug from volunteers following the bolus or infusion of the drug in question.

Using propofol as an example, this drug conforms best to the three-compartment model. Numerous algorithms have been developed, but all rely on commencing with a bolus dose that is calculated to fill the central compartment, followed by a variable infusion rate that is equal to the redistribution of the drug between all three compartments. This is achieved through three superimposed infusions, one at a constant rate to replace drug elimination from the central compartment, and two exponentially decreasing infusions to match drug that redistributes to the peripheral compartments.

It should be noted that all of the models rely on complex mathematical algorithms that are usually patented to the various manufacturers, and can only make an estimate of the true pharmacokinetics of the drug.

Loading dose and maintenance dose

Loading dose equation: $LD = V_d \times C_p$

Maintenance dose equation: $Rate_{in} = Cl \times C_p$

Definition of terms used

LD = loading dose
V_d = initial volume of distribution
C_p = required peak plasma concentration
$Rate_{in}$ = rate at which drug is administered
Cl = clearance

Units

Dose of drug, usually in mg or μg.

Explanation

Patients are often given drugs by intravenous infusion. A loading dose is given in order to attain a desired drug concentration rapidly, as opposed to waiting for a longer period of time from a constant rate intravenous infusion reaching a steady-state level. It is estimated by multiplying the concentration required (C_p), by the volume of distribution (V_d). In practice, this is estimated using the patient's parameters such as gender, weight and height.

Once a steady state has been achieved, we can maintain its level if drug input equals drug output. In this case, the frequency at which maintenance doses are administered is dependent on the rate at which the drug is removed from the plasma.

As we know that the rate of output is equal to elimination, which in turn is equal to clearance multiplied by plasma concentration, we can say that to keep plasma levels stable at a steady state:

$$Rate_{in} = Cl \times C_p$$

Once the steady state has been reached, sometimes a bolus dose can be given if a higher concentration is rapidly required during the infusion. The dose can be calculated as follows:

Bolus dose = $(C_{new} - C_{actual}) \times V_p$

Clinical application/worked example

1. *A patient in the intensive care unit requires theophylline to treat their severe asthma. Calculate the loading dose required.*

Desired $C_p = 14.1\,mg/l$

$V_d = 25$ litres

Loading dose (*LD*) = $V_d \times C_p$

= 25 × 14.1

= 353 mg

2. *Give examples of other drugs in the critical environment that make use of the equations above.*

- Digoxin.
- Vancomycin.
- Phenytoin.
- Propofol.
- Remifentanil.

NB: Propofol and remifentanil are often administered by target-controlled infusion (TCI), which uses more complex pharmacokinetic calculations.

Exponential function and rate constant

$$\frac{dC}{dt} \propto C$$

Or

$$\frac{dC}{dt} = -kC$$

Definition of terms used

dC = change in concentration
dt = change in time
C = concentration
$-k$ = constant of proportionality

Units

None.

Explanation

The characteristic of an exponential relationship is that the rate at which the dependent variable, i.e. concentration (C) changes, is determined by the value of that variable at any given time. In the case of drug elimination, this means that a constant fraction of drug is removed per unit time, and the shape of the decline in concentration with time is therefore exponential.

For any given substance, the constant of proportionality (k) for this relationship is known as the **rate constant**, and for drug elimination the **elimination rate constant**. The larger the rate constant, the quicker the decline in concentration.

'$-$'k is used in this equation, as it relates to the decreasing rate of change occurring over time, as evident from wash-out or wash-in curves. Without the minus sign, the rate constant relates to an increasing rate of change over time, such as that which is evident in a positive exponential growth curve.

The elimination rate constant depends on two parameters, the volume of plasma cleared per unit time, clearance (*Cl*), and the volume to be cleared volume of distribution (*V_d*). Therefore, it may be calculated from:

$$k = \frac{Cl}{V_d}$$

Furthermore, it may be related to half-life (*t_{1/2}*) through the formula:

$$k = 0.693/t_{1/2}$$

where $0.693 = \ln(2)$ or $\log_e(2)$.

Clinical application/worked example

1. *Describe the shape of a negative exponential curve, and describe why it takes that shape.*

A negative exponential curve displays a steep upper portion that gradually plateaus off as time progresses along the *x*-axis. It is this shape because the rate at which the dependent variable changes over time is determined by the value of that variable at any one time. At high concentrations we get a high rate of change (thus the gradient of the line is steep), and at low concentrations we get a low rate of change (hence the curve plateaus off). At all times a constant fraction of drug is removed per unit time.

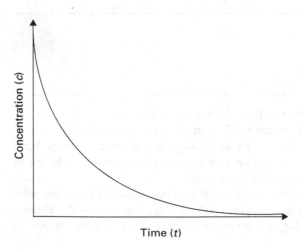

2. *An antiepileptic drug used to control seizures has a half-life of 8 hours. The drug is effective if the patient has more than 25 mg of medicine in his body. If a person takes an initial dose of 175 mg of medicine, will the medicine still be effective 24 hours later?*

If '$m(t)$' represents the quantity of medicine after 't' half lives, and 'm_o' represents the initial dose of medicine.

After 24 hours, t = 24 hours/8 hours = 3 half-lives have elapsed.

$$m(t) = m_o(0.5)^t$$

so

$$m(3) = 175(0.5)^3$$
$$m(3) = 21.88 \text{ mg}$$

Therefore, the medicine is no longer effective after 24 hours.

Half-life and context-sensitive half-life

$t_{1/2} = 0.693/k$

Or

$t_{1/2} = (0.693 \times Vd)/Cl$

Definition of terms used

$t_{1/2}$ = half-life
$0.693 = \ln(2)$ or $\log_e(2)$
V_d = volume of distribution
Cl = clearance
k = elimination rate constant

Units

Time = minutes.

Explanation

Half-life is the time taken for the plasma concentration of a drug to fall to 50% of its initial value. It governs both the time to eliminate a single dose of a drug, and the time taken for a drug to accumulate to a steady-state level during a constant rate infusion or multiple dosing regimes. This is approximately five half-lives and is normally determined experimentally.

Context-sensitive half-time (CSHT) is defined as the time taken for blood plasma concentration of a drug to fall by 50%, after an infusion designed to maintain a steady state, has been stopped. The CSHT is equal to the elimination half-life, where context refers to the duration of the infusion.

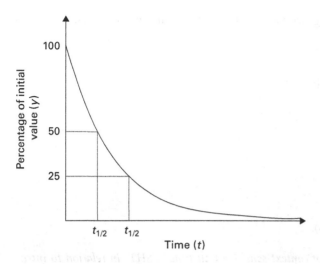

Half-life depends on the elimination rate constant (k), which is the rate at which the drug is removed from the body, and therefore may also be expressed using clearance (*Cl*) and volume of distribution (V_d) (refer to page 53).

Additionally, half-life is related to the time constant (τ) by a constant of proportionality, where ln(2) equals 0.693 (refer to page 71).

$$t_{1/2} = 0.693 \times \tau$$

From this equation, we can clearly see that the half-life is shorter than the time constant.

Clinical application/worked example

1. Demonstrate how much drug would be eliminated after five half-lives.

The half-life is the time taken for plasma concentration to fall to 50% of its initial value. The volume of plasma remaining will diminish in the following manner:

1 half-life = 50% remaining
2 half-lives = 25% remaining
3 half-lives = 12.5% remaining
4 half-lives = 6.25% remaining
5 half-lives = 3.125% remaining

After 5 half-lives approximately 97% of the drug will have been eliminated. This equates to approximately 3 time constants.

2. Give examples of drugs with long, intermediate and short half-lives.

Short
- Adenosine (< 10 s).
- Norepinephrine (2 min).

Intermediate
- Salbutamol (2–3 h).
- Morphine (2–3 h).

Long
- Diazepam (20–100 h).
- Digoxin (24–36 h).
- Amiodarone (58 days).

3. Explain the concept of context-sensitive half-time (CSHT) in relation to intra-venous infusions.

In clinical anaesthesia, drugs such as propofol, remifentanil, fentanyl and alfentanil are commonly administered by intravenous (iv) infusions. Once the infusions are stopped, two possible processes cause a drop in plasma concentration: re-distribution and excretion. The time taken for the concentration to halve will depend on the pharmacokinetics of the drug, and the length of the infusion: this determines the 'context' in this case.

The drugs have very different CSHTs and also different patterns of changes as the infusion time increases. For example, the CSHT of propofol varies between 3 min for a very short infusion to about 18 min after a 12-h infusion. The success of remifentanil is attributed to the fact that it is relatively context-**in**sensitive, whereas fentanyl has a CSHT of about 50 min after 2 h of infusion and approximately 250 min after 6 h.

Time constant

$\tau = 1/k$

Or

$\tau = V_d/Cl$

Definition of terms used

τ = time constant
k = rate constant
V_d = volume of distribution
Cl = clearance

Units

Time = minutes.

Explanation

In a single-compartment model, there is a single exponential relationship between plasma concentration and time that is governed by the rate constant (refer to page 65).

The time constant, calculated as the inverse of the rate constant, expresses how quickly the plasma concentration will fall. It is defined as the time it would have taken the plasma concentration to fall to zero if the original rate of elimination had continued.

Mathematically, the time constant is the time taken for the plasma concentration to fall from the concentration at time zero (C_0) to C/e, where e is Euler's number. By this calculation, in one time constant the plasma concentration will fall to 37% of its original value. By comparison, half-life, the time taken for concentration to fall from C_0 to $C/2$, will see a 50% fall in plasma concentration (refer to page 68).

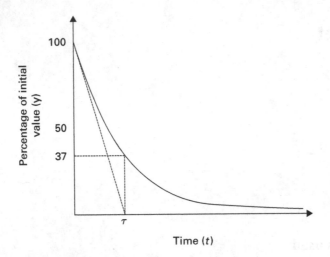

The time constant may also be calculated from its relationship to clearance (*Cl*) and volume of distribution (V_d).

$$\tau = \frac{V_d}{Cl}$$

Clinical application/worked example

1. Describe the difference between the half-life and time constant of a drug.

Time constant is defined as the time it would have taken the plasma concentration to fall to zero if the original rate of elimination had continued.

Half-life is the time taken for the plasma concentration of a drug to fall to 50% of its initial value.

Rates of reaction

$$\text{Zero order: } \frac{dA}{dt} = -k^*$$

$$\text{First order: } \frac{dA}{dt} = -kA$$

Definition of terms used

dA = change in concentration of drug A
dt = change in time
$-k^*$ = zero-order rate constant
$-kA$ = first-order rate constant

Units

Rate constant units are mg/min.

Explanation

The rate of reaction describes the speed at which a process ensues. It may be described as zero order or first order. It is commonly referred to when discussing the elimination of drugs from the body.

A **zero-order reaction**, otherwise known as saturation kinetics, describes a reaction that proceeds at a constant rate irrespective of the concentration of drug in the body. It indicates the enzyme activity is maximal.
Plotted, concentration versus time gives a straight line

A **first-order reaction** describes a reaction that proceeds at a rate which is dependent on the concentration of the drug in question. At each moment in time, a constant fraction of drug is eliminated.
Plotted, concentration versus time gives a straight line.

The equations reflect the differences described because first-order reactions include 'A' within the equation whereas the equation for zero-order reactions does not, as the rate of the reaction is independent of the drug concentration.

The metabolism of most drugs used in clinical practice is first-order as there is normally a relative abundance of enzyme (and thus enzyme activity) as compared to substrate (the drug or its metabolites). This said, if given in large enough quantities, enzyme pathways can become saturated, and virtually all drugs will eventually change from a first-order to zero-order process.

Clinical application/worked example

1. *Give examples of zero-order and first-order kinetics, and briefly describe their pharmacokinetics.*

(i) **Ethanol**: the rate-limiting step in its metabolism by alcohol dehydrogenase is the presence of a co-factor which is only present in small quantities. Importantly, in zero-order reactions, no steady state is reached, accumulation occurs, and thus a small increase in dose administered may produce a large increase in plasma concentration.

(ii) **Thiopentone**: the primary site of metabolism is in the liver. Hepatic clearance has a low hepatic extraction ratio and capacity-dependent elimination that is influenced by hepatic enzyme activity. When low doses are used, e.g. a single induction dose of 5 mg/kg for induction of anaesthesia, then first-order kinetics results. If large doses or an intravenous infusion is used, then the hepatic enzymes are saturated and zero-order kinetics result with an associated increase in elimination half-life. (Others: phenytoin, high-dose salicylates.)

(iii) **Propofol**: metabolism always undergoes first-order kinetics. As you increase the dose administered, the rate of elimination increases accordingly. A steady state will be reached, and thus accumulation will not occur.

Michaelis–Menten equation

$$V = \frac{V_{max}[s]}{K_m + [s]}$$

Definition of terms used

V = velocity of reaction (i.e. the rate at which an enzyme can metabolize its substrate)

V_{max} = maximum velocity of reaction

$[s]$ = substrate concentration

K_m = substrate concentration at which the velocity of the reaction (V) is half maximal velocity (Michaelis constant)

Units

Michaelis constant (K_m) = mmol/l
Velocity = m/s
Substrate concentration = mmol/l

Explanation

The Michaelis–Menten (Leonor Michaelis, Maud Menten 1913) model of enzyme kinetics describes the rate of an enzymatic reaction (V) whereby a single substrate (s) reacts with a single enzyme (e) via an intermediate complex (es) to produce a single product (p):

$s + e \leftrightarrow es \leftrightarrow p$

The equation illustrates the dependence of the rate of an enzyme reaction on substrate concentration, and from this, it allows one to predict which order of reaction will occur.

In simple terms,

(1) When [s] ≪ K_m, [s] can be discounted, thus:

$$V = \frac{V_{max}[s]}{K_m}$$

In this instance, as the rate and substrate concentrations are directly proportional to each other, the reaction is **first-order kinetics** (refer to page 73).

(2) When [s] ≫ K_m, K_m can be discounted, [s] consequently cancels out, thus:

$$V = V_{max}$$

In this instance, as the rate is equal to the maximum velocity and independent of the substrate concentration, the reaction is **zero-order kinetics** (refer to page 73).

The Michaelis constant is also the inverse of the affinity of substrate for an enzyme. In other words, a small K_m indicates a high affinity meaning that V_{max} will be approached quickly, and the inverse is also true. The value of K_m is also dependent on the conditions in which the enzymatic reaction occurs, such as temperature and pH.

In order to determine the constants in the equation, a series of enzyme assays are run in the laboratory at various concentrations of substrate. The reaction rate is measured at time 0 and then reaction rate can be plotted against [s]. Using non-linear regression of the Michaelis–Menten equation, V_{max} and K_m can be obtained.

Clinical application/worked example

1. Describe the kinetics of phenytoin using the terms of the Michaelis–Menten equation.

Phenytoin elimination shows mixed-order kinetic behaviour. Initially when the concentration is low, $[s] \ll K_m$, and therefore from the above we can see that rate is directly proportional to substrate concentration, and first order kinetics is evident.

As the concentrations of phenytoin increase in the blood, the metabolizing enzymes become saturated, $[s] \gg K_m$. Therefore, the rate of reaction is equal to maximal velocity (V_{max}) and consequently the reaction is zero-order.

Drug–receptor dissociation constant and affinity

$$K_d = \frac{[D][R]}{[DR]}$$

$$\text{Affinity} = \frac{1}{K_d}$$

Definition of terms used

K_d = dissociation constant
D = drug (sometimes stated as a Ligand [L])
R = receptor

Units

Molar units [M].

Explanation

The dissociation constant K_d, determined experimentally, is defined as 'the concentration of drug $[D]$ at which half of the receptors are occupied'.

If we take the simple example of where drug (D) is in close proximity to a receptor (R), at any one time D can be free of R, or bound together (DR).

$D + R \Leftrightarrow DR$

At the point of equilibrium, the proportion of receptors in each state (bound or unbound) is dependent on the dissociation constant (K_d). It therefore measures the propensity of the bound complex to dissociate into its components and so is the inverse of the association constant (although this is not often referred to in clinical pharmacology).

K_d is an intrinsic property of any drug–receptor interaction, and it is used to describe a drugs affinity for a receptor. The affinity, calculated as the reciprocal of K_d, describes how tightly a drug binds to its receptor. The smaller the dissociation constant, the larger the affinity and the stronger the drug–receptor binding. High-affinity binding will occur at low drug concentrations and low-affinity binding at high concentrations. This explains why affinity is the reciprocal of the dissociation constant.

Note that pKa is the particular dissociation constant for acid–base reactions (refer to page 157).

Clinical application/worked example

1. How does the concept of drug–receptor affinity apply to non-depolarizing muscle relaxants?

Non-depolarizing muscle relaxants (NDMRs) bind to the nicotinic receptors of the neuromuscular junction (NMJ) and cause receptor antagonism. The NMDRs have varied affinity for the cholinergic binding sites and this, in general, can be predicted by the Bowman principle: that is, weaker antagonists at the NMJ have a more rapid onset of action as they are given in a higher dose for the same effect.

For example, vecuronium has about 5 times the affinity of rocuronium and is therefore given in a dose that is 5 times the dose of vecuronium to achieve the same effect.

2. Describe how knowledge of affinity can help in the design of new drugs.

Pharmaceutical researchers can manipulate the affinity of drugs for particular protein targets. Because drugs often produce their unwanted side effects through their interaction with receptors with which they were not designed to interact, research is aimed at either designing drugs that have a high affinity for their target protein, or at improving the affinity between a particular drug and its desired receptor.

Therapeutic index

$$T_I = \frac{TD_{50}}{ED_{50}}$$

Definition of terms used

T_I = therapeutic index

TD_{50} = toxic dose: the dose of drug that causes a toxic response in 50% of the population

ED_{50} = effective dose: the dose of drug that is therapeutically effective in 50% of the population.

Units

Fraction.

Explanation

The therapeutic index refers to the relationship between a particular drug's toxic and therapeutic dose. It is calculated as the ratio between the two, the latter being the dose that produces a clinically desired or effective response.

In animal studies, the toxic dose (TD_{50}) may be substituted for the lethal dose (LD_{50}) – the dose of drug that causes death in 50% of the population.

Clinical application/worked example

1. *Give examples of drugs that have a narrow or wide therapeutic index, and describe the concerns related to this.*

Warfarin (2:1), digoxin (2:1) and gentamicin (2:1) all have a narrow therapeutic index. Remifentanil (33,000:1) and diazepam (100:1) have wide therapeutic indices.

For drugs with a narrow therapeutic index, small differences in the dose administered or plasma concentration may have serious adverse events. This may be considered so serious that daily blood tests are warranted in order to calculate the daily dose administered.

Conversely, drugs with a wider therapeutic index are regarded as more giving; however, this does not account for the fact that drugs such as remifentanil can have lethal side effects such as apnoea even within 'safe' doses.

To overcome this, another term is used to denote the safety of the drug: margin of safety (MOS). To calculate this, a ratio is taken of the dose that is just within the lethal range (LD_{01}) to the dose that is 99% effective (ED_{99}). If the MOS is less than 1, extreme caution should be taken.

Cardiac output and cardiac index

$$CO = HR \times SV$$

And

$$CI = \frac{CO}{BSA}$$

Definition of terms used

CO = cardiac output (otherwise stated as Q or Qc)
HR = heart rate
SV = stroke volume
CI = cardiac index
BSA = body surface area

Units

$CO = l/min.$

Normal adult resting value $= 4.5–5.5\,l/min.$

$CI = l/min/m^2.$

Normal adult resting value $2.6–4.2\,l/min/m^2.$

Explanation

Cardiac output is the volume of blood pumped per minute by each ventricle of the heart. The cardiac output is principally determined by the stroke volume (refer to page 83) and the heart rate, and thus alterations in either of these parameters will change the cardiac output.

Increased cardiac output is predominantly attributed to an increase in heart rate (which can vary by a factor of approximately three), while alterations in stroke volume (which can vary between 70 and 120 ml) play a lesser part. This is particularly true in children.

Cardiac output may be calculated using the Fick principle (refer to page 92); however, in routine clinical practice, it is routinely measured using a number of methods such as transoesophageal Doppler, pulse contour analysis or echocardiography.

Cardiac index is simply the relationship of cardiac output to body surface area. Cardiac index enables an assessment of ventricular function independently of body size. It therefore more accurately relates heart performance to the individual.

Clinical application/worked example

1. *A patient is administered 3 mg of atropine. How will this alter their cardiac output?*

Atropine is an anticholinergic drug, whose predominant effects would be to increase the patient's heart rate. An increase in heart rate would cause a consequent increase in cardiac output.

2. *How can knowledge of the cardiac output equation be used in clinical anaesthetic practice?*

Cardiac output monitors are routinely used during anaesthesia for major surgery to guide the response to fluids. For example, if the cardiac output is found to be lower than normal, a fluid challenge can be given and the resulting effects on the stroke volume can be monitored. If stroke volume increases, this will have a proportional effect on the cardiac output. If the stroke volume remains unchanged and the heart rate is normal, then it is likely that the low cardiac output is unrelated to the filling status of the ventricles.

Stroke volume

$SV = EDV - ESV$

Definition of terms used

SV = stroke volume
EDV = end diastolic volume
ESV = end systolic volume

Units

ml.

Normal in 70 kg man = 70–80 ml (range 55–100 ml).

Explanation

The stroke volume is the volume ejected from the ventricle with each myocardial contraction. It may be estimated using an echocardiogram, by subtracting the volume of blood in the ventricle pre- (EDV) and post- (ESV) contraction, or by pulse contour analysis.

Stroke volume is dependent on the heart rate, contractility, preload and afterload, and knowledge of Starling's law of the heart is fundamental to its understanding: *The energy of contraction of a cardiac muscle fibre, like that of a skeletal muscle fibre, is proportional to the initial fibre length at rest.*

Stroke volume is also used to calculate the ejection fraction (see page 87).

In a similar manner to cardiac index (refer to page 81), stroke volume index may be used to relate stroke volume to an individual's size.

$SVI = SV/BSV$

Clinical application/worked example

1. Give some examples of how stroke volume may be altered.

Stroke volume is determined by subtracting the volume of blood in the ventricle pre- and post-contraction, thus any factor that alters these two dynamics will increase or decrease stroke volume. These may include:

(i)   Tachycardia decreases diastolic time; thus, there is less time to fill the ventricle and consequently preload is decreased.
(ii) Fluid boluses increase preload and EDV, thus increasing stroke volume.
(iii) Aortic stenosis increases afterload, thus decreasing stroke volume.
(iv) Dobutamine, a positive inotrope, increases contractility therefore stroke volume increases.

Ventricular stroke work and index

$$LVSW = SV \times (MSAP - LAP) \times 0.0136$$
$$RVSW = SV \times (MPAP - RAP) \times 0.0136$$

Definition of terms used

$LVSW$ = left ventricular stroke work
$RVSW$ = right ventricular stroke work
SV = stroke volume
$MSAP$ = mean systemic artery pressure
$MPAP$ = mean pulmonary artery pressure
LAP = left atrial pressure (= pulmonary capillary wedge pressure)
RAP = right atrial pressure
Both equations can be indexed (LVSWI and RVSWI) to body surface area (BSA) by substituting SVI (stroke volume index) for SV.

Units

LVSW and RVSW: cJ (centi Joules)
LVSWI and RVSWI: cJ/m^2

Explanation

The stroke work describes the work done by each ventricle to eject a volume (stroke volume) of blood and is used as a surrogate for contractility. The force applied to the volume of blood is the intraventricular pressure, which as kinetic energy is assumed to be negligible, is substituted for:
(1) mean systolic aortic pressure (afterload) minus left atrial pressure (preload) in the case of the left ventricle, and
(2) mean pulmonary artery pressure minus right atrial pressure in the case of the right ventricle.
The factor 0.0136 is used to convert pressure and volume to units of work.

A pressure–volume diagram is used to depict stroke work, designated by the area within the pressure–volume loop.

Clinical application/worked example

1. *Calculate the stroke work of the left ventricle given that:*

   $SV = 70\,ml$
   $MSAP = 100\,mmHg$
   $LAP = 10\,mmHg$

   LVSW = SV × (MPAP − RAP) × 0.0136
   LVSW = 70 × (100 − 10) × 0.0136
   = 85.6 cJ

Ejection fraction and fractional area change

$$EF = SV - EDV$$

And

$$FAC = \frac{(EDA - ESA)}{EDA}$$

Definition of terms used

EF = ejection fraction
SV = stroke volume
EDV = end diastolic volume
FAC = fractional area change
EDA = end diastolic area
ESA = end systolic area

Units

Percentage (%)
Normal $EF > 55\%$
Normal $FAC > 35\%$

Explanation

The ejection fraction is the volumetric fraction of blood ejected from the ventricle with each contraction. As stroke volume is calculated from end diastolic volume minus end systolic volume, the equation may be given as:

$$EF = \frac{(EDV - ESV)}{EDV}$$

Ejection fraction is commonly used as a prognostic indicator in acute and chronic heart failure, although having a preserved ejection fraction does not mean freedom from risk.

An alternative method used to assess left ventricular function is to calculate fractional area change (FAC) using echocardiography. This utilizes manual planimetry of the area circumscribed by the endocardium at end diastole (EDA) and end systole (*ESA*) to calculate *FAC*. It may be two- or three-dimensional depending on the level of echocardiography available.

Clinical application/worked example

1. Describe what happens to the ejection fraction in congestive cardiac failure (CCF).

CCF is the inability of the heart to maintain adequate perfusion of the tissues. As the ventricle becomes less efficient, usually as a result of dilation (refer to Laplace's law, page 24), the force of contraction decreases. As a result, the *EDV* increases and so ejection fraction decreases.

Coronary perfusion pressure and coronary blood flow

CPP = ADP − LVEDP

And

CBF = CPP/CVR

Definition of terms used

CPP = coronary perfusion pressure
ADP = aortic diastolic pressure
LVEDP = left ventricular end diastolic pressure
CBF = coronary blood flow
CVR = coronary vascular resistance

Units

mmHg.

Explanation

Coronary perfusion pressure refers to the pressure gradient that drives coronary blood flow, thus the two equations are closely interlinked. Notably in the case of the left ventricle, it is the diastolic pressure that is the important determination of coronary perfusion. In systole, the myocardial blood vessels are compressed and twisted by the cardiac contractions, and blood flow is negligible. These phasic changes are less pronounced on the right side, due to lesser forces of contraction.

Coronary blood flow is typically 250 ml/min (0.8 ml/min/g of heart muscle) in a 70 kg adult at rest, representing 5% of cardiac output. As cardiac arterial oxygen extraction is 80% (cf. 25% for the rest of the body), increased oxygen consumption must be met by an increase in coronary blood flow, which may increase fivefold during exercise. The equation is analogous to the electrical equation $V = IR$ (refer to Ohm's law, page 28), and allows us to see why any increase in coronary vascular resistance can lead to devastating effects.

Clinical application/worked example

1. Describe the effects of aortic stenosis and atherosclerosis on coronary blood flow.

Severe aortic stenosis, in creating an outflow obstruction to the left ventricle, results in lower aortic diastolic pressures. Referring to the equation, this in turn will decrease coronary perfusion pressures – an important determinant in coronary blood flow.

Atherosclerotic plaques on coronary blood vessels cause increased coronary vascular resistance, consequently decreasing coronary blood flow and ultimately resulting in areas of myocardial ischaemia.

2. How does left ventricular failure impact on CPP?

When the left ventricle starts to fail, there is a decrease in the proportion of blood ejected during systole (ejection fraction – refer to page 87), which in turn results in an increase in LVEDP. Using the equation, it is easy to see how CPP and CBF may fall as a result. Initially, CBP may be ameliorated by reflex systemic vaso-constriction, but this will result in an increase in pressure load and oxygen demand.

Bazett's formula – QT interval corrected

$$QTc = \frac{QT}{\sqrt{RR}}$$

Definition of terms used

QTc = QT interval corrected
QT = QT interval
RR = RR interval

Units

Time = ms.

Normal: 380–430 ms.

Explanation

The QT interval is a measure of the time in a cardiac contraction cycle, between the start of the Q wave and the end of the T wave. It represents electrical depolarization and repolarization of the ventricles.

The QT interval varies depending on the heart rate. Should the heart rate increase, the QT interval decreases and therefore various methods have been suggested to calculate a variable which is independent of the heart rate (QTc). The most common one used in clinical practice is Bazett's (Henry Cuthbert Bazett, 1920) formula, which standardizes the heart rate to 60 bpm. Others include Sagie's (Alex Sagie, 1992) formula and Fridercia's (Louis Sigurd Fridercia, 1920) formula.

Clinical application/worked example

1. *Discuss the importance of calculating the QT interval.*

A prolonged QT interval can predispose patients to ventricular arrhythmias such as torsades de pointes. It may be secondary to genetic causes (long QT syndrome), adverse drug reactions (haloperidol, amiodarone) and pathological conditions (hypothyroidism).

The Fick principle – cardiac output measurement

$$CO = \frac{VO_2}{C_aO_2 - C_vO_2}$$

Definition of terms used

CO = cardiac output
VO_2 = oxygen consumption (ml/min)
C_aO_2 = arterial oxygen concentration
C_vO_2 = venous oxygen concentration

Units

l/min.

Explanation

The Fick principle (Adolf Eugen Fick, 1870), otherwise known as the 'Inverse Fick equation', allows the measurement of cardiac output. Its underlying principle is that the blood flow to an organ can be calculated using an indicator material if we know:

(1) the amount of indicator material taken up by the organ per unit time;
(2) the concentration of indicator material in the arterial blood supplying (entering) the organ; and
(3) the concentration of indicator material in the venous blood leaving the organ.

In this case, the indicator is oxygen, and so the Fick principle can be usefully applied in normal clinical practice.

Initially, Fick's equation was used to calculate oxygen consumption in the lungs (see below), but because pulmonary blood flow is equal to right ventricular output, the equation can be rearranged to give cardiac output as above.

Clinical application/worked example

1. *At rest, an individual's oxygen consumption is 250 ml/min. Given that $C_aO_2 = 200\,ml/l$ and $C_vO_2 = 150\,ml/l$, calculate the cardiac output for this individual.*

$$CO = \frac{VO_2}{C_aO_2 - C_vO_2}$$

$$CO = 250 - (200 - 150)$$

$$= 5\,l/min$$

Derivation

Derived from the original Fick's equation.

$$VO_2 = CO \times (C_a - C_v)$$

Per unit time:

(1) *amount of oxygen entering the lungs in venous blood*

$$= CO \times C_vO_2$$

(2) *amount of oxygen leaving the lungs in arterial blood*

$$= CO \times C_aO_2$$

(3) *amount of oxygen uptake by blood as it passes through the lungs is the difference between arterial and venous concentrations*

$$= (CO \times C_aO_2) - (CO \times C_vO_2)$$

(4) *in steady state, oxygen uptake by pulmonary blood flow is equal to the removal of alveolar oxygen:*

$$VO_2 = (CO \times C_aO_2) - (CO \times C_vO_2)$$

(5) *and rearranged:*

$$VO_2 = CO \times (C_aO_2 - C_vO_2)$$

(6) *therefore:*

$$CO = \frac{VO_2}{C_aO_2 - C_vO_2}$$

The Fick equation – oxygen uptake measurement

$$VO_2 = CO \times (C_aO_2 - C_vO_2)$$

Definition of terms used

CO = cardiac output
VO_2 = oxygen consumption (ml/min)
C_aO_2 = arterial oxygen concentration
C_vO_2 = venous oxygen concentration

Units

ml/min.

Explanation

The Fick equation (Adolf Eugen Fick, 1870) tells us the rate of oxygen uptake from alveolar gas. Under aerobic conditions, oxygen is consumed to generate energy, thus VO_2 corresponds to metabolic rate. VO_{2max} (maximal oxygen uptake) is the maximal capacity of an individual to utilize oxygen. It is reached when oxygen consumption remains at a steady state despite an increase in workload.

VO_2 can be directly measured using the analysis of respiratory gases (as seen in cardiopulmonary exercise testing), or derived from cardiac output and arterial-venous oxygen contents.

The concept for VO_2 was first purported in 1870, when Fick stated that the rate at which the circulation absorbs oxygen from the lungs, must equal the change in oxygen concentration in the pulmonary blood multiplied by pulmonary blood flow.

NB: As pulmonary blood flow is equal to right ventricular output, the equation can be rearranged to give cardiac output (see Fick principle for cardiac output page 192).

Clinical application/worked example

1. Describe a use for cardiopulmonary exercise testing relating it to this equation.

Cardiopulmonary exercise testing (CPET) allows a non-invasive measurement of VO_2 and VO_{2max}. It may be used to assess the adequacy of oxygen delivery (DO_2), on the assumption that if oxygen delivery is inadequate for the demand, VO_2 becomes supply-dependent. In health, oxygen delivery matches oxygen uptake. However, if oxygen delivery decreases past the point where an increased oxygen extraction can compensate, cellular metabolic activity becomes limited by the supply of oxygen. Further reduction in oxygen delivery will result in tissue hypoxia, anaerobic metabolism and the production of lactic acid. This point may be calculated using CPET.

Derivation

Per unit time:

(1) amount of oxygen entering lungs in venous blood

$$= CO \times C_v O_2$$

(2) amount of oxygen leaving lungs in arterial blood

$$= CO \times C_a O_2$$

(3) amount of oxygen uptake by blood as it passes through the lungs is the difference between arterial and venous concentrations

$$= (CO \times C_a O_2) - (CO \times C_v O_2)$$

(4) in steady state, oxygen uptake by pulmonary blood flow is equal to the removal of alveolar oxygen:

$$VO_2 = (CO \times C_a O_2) - (CO \times C_v O_2)$$

(5) and rearranged:

$$VO_2 = CO \times (C_a O_2 - C_v O_2)$$

Mean arterial pressure

$$MAP = (CO \times SVR) + CVP$$

Definition of terms used

MAP = mean arterial pressure
CO = cardiac output
SVR = systemic vascular resistance
CVP = central venous pressure

Units

mmHg.

Explanation

The mean arterial pressure, in an analogous manner to electricity (refer to Ohm's law, page 28), is based upon the relationship between pressure (V), flow (I) and resistance (R) ($V = I \times R$). As CVP is usually near to 0 mmHg, the equation is often simplified to:

$$MAP = CO \times SVR.$$

In routine clinical practice, MAP is not determined using the equation as knowledge of a patient's CO and SVR are often not to hand, but rather using measurements of blood pressure.

From the assessment of an arterial pressure trace over time, approximately 2/3 of the cardiac cycle is spent in diastole. Therefore, the mean pressure value (geometric mean) is lower than the calculated arithmetic mean of the diastolic and systolic pressures. Note that if there is a tachycardia the equation may change nearing to the arithmetic mean of half the pulse pressure + the diastolic pressure.

At normal heart rates, *MAP* can therefore be approximated using the following equations.

$$MAP = DBP + \frac{1}{3}PP$$

where *DBP* = diastolic blood pressure; *SBP* = systolic blood pressure; *PP* = pulse pressure.

Clinical application/worked example

1. *A septic patient on the intensive care unit has a blood pressure of 82/37 mmHg and a heart rate of 75 bpm. Approximate their mean arterial pressure.*

Pulse pressure = *SBP* − *DBP*

= 82 − 37

= 45 mmHg

Mean arterial pressure = DBP + (1/3 × PP)

= 37 + (1/3 × 45)

= 52 mmHg

2. *Describe what would happen if noradrenaline was administered to the patient.*

Noradrenaline is predominantly a vasopressor. Its administration would increase *SVR*, and assuming that the *CO* remained the same, the patient's *MAP* would increase.

Venous return

$$VR = \frac{P_V - P_{RA}}{R_V}$$

Definition of terms used

VR = venous return
P_V = venous pressure
P_{RA} = right atrial pressure
R_V = venous resistance

Units

ml/min.

Explanation

Haemodynamically, venous return to the heart from peripheral venous vascular beds is determined by a pressure gradient ($P_V - P_{RA}$) and the venous resistance. Therefore, any action that increases venous pressure, or decreases right atrial pressure or venous resistance, will increase venous return.

The equation for venous return is analogous to Ohm's law of '$V = IR$' (refer to page 28), where:

$V = P_V - P_{RA}$

$I = VR$ and

$R = R_V$

As the cardiovascular system is a closed loop, the venous return must equal cardiac output. This is balanced by the Frank–Starling mechanism. However, while both are interdependent, each can be independently regulated.

Clinical application/worked example

1. Give examples of factors that influence venous return.

(i) Deep inspiration, such as that of the valsava manoeuvre, increases resistance in the thoracic vena cava, and thus decreases venous return (VR).

(ii) Decreased venous compliance (due to increased sympathetic activity) increases central venous pressure and promotes venous return indirectly by augmenting cardiac output through the Frank–Starling mechanism.

(iii) Laparoscopic surgery and gross insufflation of the abdomen compresses the abdominal vena cava, and thus decreases venous return through increased R_V. This causes a detrimental effect on cardiac output.

Total blood volume

$$TBV = \frac{V_p}{1 - Hct}$$

Or rearranged

$$TBV = \frac{V_p \times 100}{100 - Hct}$$

Definition of terms used

TBV = total blood volume
V_p = plasma volume
Hct = haematocrit

Units

ml or l.

Normal adult range: 4.5–5.5 l.

Explanation

Total blood volume can be indirectly determined if the plasma volume and haematocrit are known.

The plasma volume in litres can be estimated using the following equation:

$$V_p = 0.07 \times weight\,(kg) \times (1 - Hct)$$

NB: Whole body haematocrit may be overestimated, as (1) laboratory-measured haematocrit overestimates the true value as approximately 4–8% of plasma remains confined with the red cells in the tube, and (2) capillary blood has a lower haematocrit than larger vessels due to axial streaming of red blood cells.

Clinical application/worked example

1. *Calculate the plasma volume and total blood volume for this patient in the intensive care unit:*

Weight = 75 kg

Haematocrit = 0.320

V_p = 0.07 × 75 × (1 − 0.320) = 3.57 litres

TBV = 3.57/(1 − 0.320)

= 5.25 litres

Systemic vascular resistance

$$SVR = \left(\frac{MAP - CVP}{CO} \right) \times 80$$

Definition of terms used

SVR = systemic vascular resistance
MAP = mean arterial pressure
CVP = central venous pressure
CO = cardiac output

Units

dyn·s/cm^5.

Normal range 800–1600 dyn·s/cm^5.

Explanation

Otherwise referred to as total peripheral resistance, the systemic vascular resistance denotes the resistance to blood flow demonstrated by all vessels, bar the pulmonary circulation. SVR is often thought to be analogous to the afterload on the left ventricle. As central venous pressure normally approximates to 0, the equation may be simplified to:

$$SVR = \frac{MAP}{CO}$$

Importantly, although SVR is calculated from MAP and CO, it is not determined by either of these variables. While in the above equation SVR is the dependent variable, physiologically SVR and CO are the independent variables, and MAP the dependent variable.

The figure of 80 is used as a correction factor to change mmHg to dyn·s/cm^5.

SVR may be indexed (SVRI) to body surface area (BSA) by substituting CO in the equation for cardiac index (CI). Normal range is 1970–2390 dyn·s/cm^5/m^2.

Clinical application/worked example

1. What factors directly decrease and increase the SVR?

Decrease	Increase
Anaemia (through reduced viscosity)	Severe pre-eclampsia
Fever (through increased O_2 demand)	Essential hypertension
Sepsis	Smoking
Anaphylaxis	Diabetes
Most general anaesthetic agents	Obesity

2. How does knowledge of the equation assist in the management of a critically ill hypotensive patient?

Commonly, critically ill patients have a decreased *MAP*. However, it can be challenging to determine which aspects of the cardiovascular system need to be manipulated in order to restore a 'normal' blood pressure.

Knowledge of the equation, in conjunction with clinical examination and possibly a cardiac output monitor, can assist in the following manner:

CO	SVR	Conditions	Management
Low	High	Cardiogenic shock, haemorrhagic shock	Optimize fluid status, inotropy
High	Low	Sepsis	Optimize fluid status, vasoconstriction
Low	Low	Drug-induced	Correct underlying cause

Uterine blood flow

$$UBF = \frac{UP_a - UP_v}{UVR}$$

Definition of terms used

UBF = uterine blood flow
UP_a = uterine artery pressure
UP_v = uterine venous pressure
UVR = uterine vascular resistance

Units

ml/min.

Explanation

The equation for uterine blood flow is analogous to Ohm's law '$V = IR$' (refer to page 28) where:

$V = UP_a - UP_v$

$I = UBF$ and

$R = UVR$

Maintaining an adequate flow (approximately 500–700 ml/min at term) is fundamental, as the uterine blood flow supports the foeto-placental circulation upon which the developing foetus is entirely reliant. In a normal healthy placenta, uterine blood flow can decrease by about 50% before foetal distress, diagnosed by the presence of foetal acidosis, is detected.

Importantly, uterine blood flow is not autoregulated, and thus wholly reliant on the pressure gradient ($UP_a - UP_v$) and the local resistance (UVR). Any drugs that alter either of these will affect uterine blood flow.

Clinical application/worked example

1. Discuss the methods used in anaesthesia to maintain uterine blood flow.

Uterine blood flow is dependent on maintaining an adequate perfusion gradient, and minimizing uterine vascular resistance.

Methods used to achieve this are:

(i) Placing the pregnant patient in the left lateral position so as to minimize aortocaval compression (and thus decreased UP_a through decreased cardiac output).

(ii) Maintaining an adequate systemic blood pressure when performing regional anaesthesia through the administration of intravenous fluids and peripheral vasoconstrictors.

(iii) Minimizing the use of drugs that cause uterine vasoconstriction, thereby increasing UVR.

Stewart–Hamilton equation

$$CO = \left(\frac{k \times (T_{blood} - T_{injectate}) \times V_{injectate}}{\int \Delta T_B \times dt} \right)$$

Or modified to suit dye-dilution techniques:

$$CO = \frac{\text{amount of injected indicator}}{\text{area under dilution curve}}$$

Definition of terms used

CO = cardiac output
$V_{injectate}$ = volume of injectate
k = correction factor
T_{blood} = temperature of blood
$T_{injectate}$ = temperature of injectate
$\int \Delta T_B \times dt$ = integral of area under temperature/time curve

Units

l/min.

Explanation

There are several methods used to calculate cardiac output. The thermodilution technique utilizes the Stewart–Hamilton equation (George Neil Stewart, 1897 and William Hamilton, 1932). It is based on the principle that the cardiac output is equal to the amount of an indicator injected divided by its average concentration in the arterial blood after a single circulation through the heart.

The denominator of the equation equates to the quantity of injectate and the numerator refers to its concentration.

Clinical application/worked example

1. How is the Stewart–Hamilton equation applied to the pulmonary artery catheter?

In clinical practice, a number of indicators can be used. The gold standard remains cold saline that is injected through the proximal port of a pulmonary artery catheter (PAC). The resultant temperature change of the blood is measured by a distally positioned thermistor. Alternatively, the blood is heated proximally by cyclical heating filament. This provides serial CO measurements.

A graph of time vs. temperature change is plotted, and the above equation used to calculate CO. The cardiac output is inversely proportional to the mean blood-temperature depression and the duration of transit of cooled blood (area under the curve).

This method assumes, and is reliant on (1) constant blood flow, (2) no loss of indicator from the circulation between injection and detection, and (3) complete mixing of indicator and blood.

Oxygen delivery

$$DO_2 = CO \times ((S_aO_2 \times Hb \times 1.34) + (0.003 \times P_aO_2))$$

Simplified to

$$DO_2 = CO \times C_aO_2$$

Definition of terms used

DO_2 = oxygen flux
CO = cardiac output
S_aO_2 = saturation of haemoglobin with oxygen
Hb = haemoglobin (g/dl)
P_aO_2 = arterial partial pressure of oxygen
1.34 = oxygen carrying capacity of 1 g of haemoglobin (ml/g)
0.003 = quantity of oxygen dissolved in plasma at one atmosphere and body
    temperature (ml/dl/mmHg).
C_aO_2 = oxygen content of arterial blood.

Units

ml/min.

Explanation

As oxygen is predominantly carried by haemoglobin, its delivery (otherwise known as flux), is calculated by multiplying the oxygen content of arterial blood (refer to page 112) by the cardiac output (refer to page 81).

At present, it is only practical to routinely measure global oxygen delivery; however, if regional blood flow is available, the same principles can be used to measure local blood flow.

Clinical application/worked example

1. Discuss the factors that alter oxygen flux.

Hypoxia, the deficiency of oxygen at the tissue level, may be caused by any number of factors that affect the above equation.

(1) Decreased arterial oxygen content as a consequence of:
  (i) anaemic hypoxia – decreased oxygen carrying capacity secondary to low haemoglobin levels, or increased abnormal forms of haemoglobin that are unable to bind to oxygen;
  (ii) hypoxic hypoxia – a decrease in the amount of oxygen bound to haemoglobin;
(2) decreased cardiac output (stagnant hypoxia), normally secondary to inadequate circulating volume (hypovolaemia) or inadequate cardiac function (cardiogenic shock).

Oxygen extraction ratio

$$O_2ER = VO_2/DO_2$$

Or otherwise defined as

$$O_2ER = C_aO_2 - C_vO_2/C_aO_2$$

Definition of terms used

O_2ER = oxygen extraction ratio
C_aO_2 = arterial oxygen content
C_vO_2 = venous oxygen content
VO_2 = oxygen uptake
DO_2 = oxygen delivery (refer to page 108)

Units

Nil – it is a ratio.

Explanation

The oxygen extraction ratio is the ratio of oxygen uptake to oxygen delivery. It therefore represents the fraction of oxygen delivered to the microcirculation and taken up by the metabolizing cells. Different organs utilize different amounts of oxygen; however, globally the normal O_2ER is 0.2–0.3, i.e. 20–30% of oxygen is utilized. Organs with high extraction ratios include the heart (60%) and the brain (35%).

Clinical application/worked example

1. Describe how the oxygen extraction ratio may alter in critical illness.

In normal health, systemic VO_2 reflects the body's metabolic demands and remains relatively independent of DO_2. In critical illness, if the DO_2 cannot match the VO_2, the increased metabolic demands will initially be met by increasing the oxygen extraction ratio.

This increase in oxygen extraction can be assessed by looking at 'mixed venous oxygen saturations' (S_vO_2), which in health would normally be above 75%. However, in situations of critical illness where the O_2ER increases, the mixed venous oxygen saturations may drop below that. This has been shown in some studies to be a poor prognostic indicator, particularly in sepsis.

Oxygen content equation

$$C_aO_2 = (S_aO_2 \times Hb \times 1.34) + (0.003 \times P_aO_2)$$

Or simplified to

$$C_aO_2 = S_aO_2 \times 1.34 \times Hb$$

Definition of terms used

C_aO_2 = arterial oxygen content
S_aO_2 = saturation of haemoglobin with oxygen (expressed as a fraction of 1.0 rather than a percentage, e.g. 0.97 instead of 97%)
Hb = haemoglobin (g/dl)
P_aO_2 = arterial partial pressure of oxygen (mmHg)
1.34 = oxygen carrying capacity of 1 g haemoglobin (ml/g)
(This may be defined as 1.39 depending on the reference and the way it is derived. This is due to the presence and binding of substances such as methaemoglobin and carboxyhaemoglobin to haemoglobin, thereby changing its conformation to one that will not bind oxygen.)
0.003 = quantity of oxygen dissolved in plasma at one atmosphere and body temperature (ml/dl/mmHg)
(The solubility of oxygen in blood is 0.03 ml/l/mmHg; however, to bring the units into agreement with others in the equation this number is divided by 10.)

Units

ml O_2/dl.

Explanation

This equation is used to describe the oxygen carrying capacity of blood. To remain viable, tissues require a certain amount of oxygen delivered per unit time – a need met by requisite oxygen content, not partial pressure.

Importantly, the amount of oxygen dissolved in plasma is generally very small relative to the haemoglobin-bound oxygen and thus in normal circumstances contributes very little to the oxygen content ($< 1.5\%$). It does, however, become very significant when the partial pressure of oxygen is increased, such as in a hyperbaric chamber, or in severe anaemia.

If haemoglobin levels are adequate, then patients can demonstrate a reduced partial pressure of oxygen and still provide sufficient oxygen delivery for the tissues. Conversely, patients can have a normal P_aO_2, and still be profoundly hypoxaemic due to (i) the altered affinity of haemoglobin to oxygen, (ii) anaemia, (iii) cytotoxicity, and (iv) hypovolaemia.

Clinical application/worked example

1. A patient in A&E has the following parameters:

Hb: 15 g/dl, SpO_2: 98%, P_aO_2: 100 mmHg.
Calculate their arterial oxygen content.

$$C_aO_2 = (S_aO_2 \times Hb \times 1.34) + (0.003 \times P_aO_2)$$
$$C_aO_2 = (0.98 \times 15 \times 1.34) + (0.003 \times 100)$$
$$= 19.7 \, \text{ml/dl}$$

2. Describe the benefit of using hyperbaric oxygen for carbon monoxide poisoning.

Carbon monoxide (CO) has a greater affinity to haemoglobin than oxygen, and consequently in the presence of CO, oxygen content decreases.

Normally the amount of dissolved oxygen in the blood contributes very little to the overall oxygen content ($< 1.5\%$); however, if a patient is subjected to increased pressures in a hyperbaric chamber, their partial pressure of oxygen increases. This in turn means that the dissolved oxygen contributes far more to the C_aO_2. If the pressure is increased from one to three atmospheres, the dissolved oxygen alone could be adequate to meet the patient's metabolic requirements.

The dilution principle – measurement of fluid compartment volume

$$V = \frac{M}{C}$$

Definition of terms used

V = volume
M = mass
C = concentration

Units

ml.

Explanation

Fluid compartment volumes are measured by determining the volume of distribution of an indicator. A known mass of indicator is added to a compartment, and after sufficient time to allow for equilibrium to be reached and uniform distribution throughout the compartment, the compartment volume is calculated from the above equation.

The indicator must be rapidly and uniformly distributed throughout only the compartment in question, and it should not be metabolized or excreted.

Clinical application/worked example

1. *Describe the methods of measuring body compartments which utilize this equation.*

   (i)   Total body water: tritium oxide (an isotope of water).
   (ii) Extracellular fluid: crystalloids (inulin, mannitol), ionics (chloride isotopes).
   (iii) Plasma volume: Evans blue (binds to albumin), radio-iodine labelled serum albumin (RISA).
   (iv) Blood volume: radio-chromium labelled red cells.

Diffusing capacity

$$D_L CO = \frac{VCO}{P_A CO}$$

Definition of terms used

$D_L CO$ = diffusing capacity of carbon monoxide
VCO = volume of carbon monoxide (CO) transferred (ml/min)
$P_A CO$ = partial pressure of CO in alveoli

Units

ml/min/mmHg.

Normal = 25 ml/min/mmHg.

Explanation

Diffusing capacity is denoted by D_L, which stands for diffusion lung, followed by the chemical species. It is also known as the transfer factor (T_L), and commonly uses the gas carbon monoxide.

The diffusing capacity is the ability of the respiratory membrane to exchange a gas between the alveoli and the pulmonary blood. It is the volume of a gas that diffuses across the membrane per minute for each mmHg partial pressure difference. For a given gradient in partial pressure of gas, the higher the diffusing capacity, the larger the amount of gas transferred into the lung per unit time.

The 'single breath method' is the commonly used test to determine diffusing capacity. Carbon monoxide is used as the gas for this test, because oxygen diffusion into the pulmonary capillaries may be perfusion-limited, whereas CO is solely diffusion-limited. Furthermore, as CO rapidly binds to haemoglobin, the partial pressure of CO in capillary blood ($P_c CO$) is negligible and can be neglected in calculations ($P_A CO - P_c CO = P_A CO$).

Clinical application/worked example

1. *A subject moderately exercising demonstrates a VCO of 40 ml/min, and an alveolar P_ACO of 0.7 mmHg. What is their diffusing capacity for CO?*

$D_LCO = 40/0.7$
$= 57$ ml/min/mmHg

2. *What gas is commonly used to measure the diffusing capacity of the lung?*

Carbon monoxide is commonly used because of the following.
 (i) Its uptake is limited by diffusion and not blood flow.
 (ii) Under normal circumstances there is essentially no CO in venous blood.
 (iii) The affinity of CO for haemoglobin is 210-times greater than that of oxygen. This means that the partial pressure of CO is essentially zero in the pulmonary capillaries.

3. *Give examples of what would cause the diffusing capacity to decrease.*

 (i) Pulmonary oedema.
 (ii) Pulmonary fibrosis.
 (iii) Emphysema.

Compliance

$$Compliance = \frac{\Delta\ volume}{\Delta\ pressure}$$

Definition of terms used

Δ Pressure = change in pressure
Δ Volume = change in volume

Units

ml/cmH_2O.
Normal total lung compliance = $100 - 200\ ml/cmH_2O$.

Explanation

Compliance describes the volume change per unit change in pressure. It is demonstrated by the slope of a pressure–volume curve. In clinical practice, it is often used to refer to the lungs or arteries.

It is important to understand the concept of compliance with regards to mechanical ventilation. Over the normal range (tidal volumes), the lung is extremely compliant; however, at very low volumes, or very high volumes, compliance decreases as the lung is stiffer. Therefore, a greater change in pressure is needed for the same change in volume.

Lungs also demonstrate hysteresis: for identical volumes, compliance is different between inspiration and expiration. Lung volume at any given pressure is larger during expiration than inflation.

Pulmonary compliance may be described as being 'static' or 'dynamic'. Static compliance describes the lung's compliance during periods with no gas flow. At this time, for example during an inspiratory pause, the effects of airway resistance are eliminated. The static compliance curve can be used to set the ideal level of PEEP (positive end expiratory pressure) for a patient undergoing mechanical ventilation. Normal values are $60-100\ ml/cmH_2O$.

Static compliance can be measured clinically using the following equation:

$$Compliance_{Static} = \frac{V_t}{Pplat - PEEP}$$

(V_t = tidal volume, P_{plat} = plateau pressure, PEEP = positive and expiratory pressure)

Dynamic compliance reflects the lung's compliance during periods of gas flow; for example, during inspiration or expiration. It is always less than or equal to static lung compliance.

The equation used to calculate the compliance for the total respiratory system (CR) is calculated from the lung compliance (Cl) and the chest wall compliance (Cw).

$$\frac{1}{CR} = \frac{1}{Cl} + \frac{1}{Cw}$$

Clinical application/worked example

1. Describe the role of surfactant in altering compliance.

Secreted by type II alveolar epithelial cells, surfactant is a phospholipid synthesized from fatty acids in the lung. Dipalmitoyl-phosphatidylcholine (DPPC) is a constituent of surfactant and due to its hydrophobic and hydrophilic nature, it opposes the normal attracting forces between liquid surface molecules which are responsible for surface tension. Decreased surface tension results in increased pulmonary compliance.

2. Give examples of pathological conditions that would cause increased or decreased compliance.

Pulmonary fibrosis, atelectasis and pulmonary oedema are associated with decreased pulmonary compliance.

Pulmonary emphysema may be associated with increased pulmonary compliance due to the loss of alveolar and elastic tissue, as is the case with a normal aging lung.

3. Calculate the static compliance of a critically ill patient from the following:

Tidal volume = 500 ml
Plateau pressure = 20 cmH$_2$O
PEEP = 5 cmH$_2$O

$$Compliance_{Static} = \frac{V_t}{Pplat - PEEP}$$

$$= 500/(20 - 5)$$

$$= 33.3 \, ml/cmH_2O$$

Bohr equation

$$\frac{V_d}{V_t} = \frac{(P_A CO_2 - P_E CO_2)}{P_A CO_2}$$

Definition of terms used

V_d = physiological dead space
V_t = tidal volume
$P_A CO_2$ = alveolar partial pressure of CO_2
$P_E CO_2$ = mixed expired partial pressure of CO_2

Units

Nil – it is a ratio.

Normal ratio of dead space to tidal volume at rest is 0.2–0.35.

Explanation

The Bohr equation (Christian Bohr, 1855–1911) is used to derive the physio-logical dead space. It is given as a ratio of dead space to tidal volume. Its derivation (see below) is based on the fact that only ventilated alveoli involved in gas exchange will produce CO_2, and none from the dead space.

'Physiological dead space' differs from 'anatomical dead space' (measured by Fowler's method) as it measures the volume of the lung that does not eliminate CO_2, and thus includes alveolar dead space. In health, however, the volumes are almost identical.

In practice, $P_a CO_2$ can be substituted for $P_A CO_2$ and end-tidal CO_2 for $P_E CO_2$ to use this equation.

Clinical application/worked example

1. *In a measurement of physiological dead space using Bohr's method, the alveolar and mixed expired PCO_2 were 5.3 and 4 kPa, respectively. What was the ratio of dead space to tidal volume?*

The Bohr equation states:

$$\frac{V_d}{V_t} = \frac{(P_ACO_2 - P_ECO_2)}{P_ACO_2}$$

Substitute into the equation such that:

$$P_ACO_2 = 5.3$$
$$P_ECO_2 = 4$$
$$(5.3 - 4)/(5.3) = 0.25.$$

Derivation

(1) *Tidal volume (V_t) is made up of alveolar volume (V_A) and dead space volume (V_d)*

$$V_t = V_A + V_d$$

And rearranging

$$V_A = V_t - V_d$$

(2) *All expired CO_2 comes only from alveolar gas*

$$V_t \times F_E = V_A \times F_A$$

(F_E = fraction of expired CO_2, F_A = alveolar fraction of CO_2).

(3) *If we substitute in*

$$V_t \times F_E = (V_t - V_d) \times F_A$$

(4) *Multiply out the brackets and rearrange*

$$V_d/V_t = (F_A - F_E)/F_A$$

(5) *Substitute fraction of CO_2 for partial pressure of the gas*

$$V_d/V_t = (P_ACO_2 - P_ECO_2)/P_ACO_2$$

NB: *As the PCO_2 in alveolar gas and arterial blood are almost the same in normal health, the equation may be written as*

$$\frac{V_d}{V_t} = \frac{(P_ACO_2 - P_ECO_2)}{P_ACO_2}$$

Alveolar ventilation equation

$$V_A = \left(\frac{VCO_2}{P_A CO_2} \right) \times k$$

Commonly rearranged to

$$P_A CO_2 = \frac{VCO_2}{V_A}$$

Definition of terms used

V_A = alveolar ventilation (l/min)
VCO_2 = CO_2 production (ml/min)
$P_A CO_2$ = alveolar partial pressure of CO_2 (mmHg)
$P_a CO_2$ = arterial partial pressure of CO_2 (mmHg)
k = constant (0.863)

(NB: $P_A CO_2$ may be replaced by $P_a CO_2$.)

Units

See definition of terms used.

Explanation

This equation is fundamental to understanding respiratory physiology. It states that alveolar partial pressure of CO_2 ($P_A CO_2$) is directly proportional to CO_2 production, and inversely proportional to alveolar ventilation. As you increase your ventilation, you decrease your $P_A CO_2$.

Alveolar and arterial PCO_2 can be assumed to be equal, although in states of severe ventilation–perfusion mismatch, this may not be the case.

The constant 0.863 is necessary to equate dissimilar units for the above terms.

Clinical application/worked example

1. *What would happen to a patient's arterial carbon dioxide if they were administered a high dose of opioids?*

A high dose of opioids would cause respiratory depression and a consequent decrease in alveolar ventilation. If CO_2 production remained equal, then we would see an increase in arterial carbon dioxide. This is one of the causes of alveolar hypoventilation, and is the main reason for increasing the F_iO_2 to patients who are receiving opiates.

Alveolar gas equation

$$P_AO_2 = P_iO_2 - (P_ACO_2/RQ)$$

Definition of terms used

P_AO_2 = alveolar partial pressure of oxygen
P_iO_2 = partial pressure of inspired oxygen
P_ACO_2 = alveolar partial pressure of carbon dioxide
RQ = respiratory quotient

NB: $P_iO_2 = F_iO_2 \times (PATM - PH_2O)$

Units

Units of pressure.

(The standard SI unit for pressure is the pascal (Pa); however, several other units are commonly used: bar, atmospheres, mmHg, cmH₂O.)

Explanation

The alveolar gas equation is used to calculate the partial pressure of oxygen in the alveoli (P_AO_2) using data that are practically measured. It is essential to understanding any P_aO_2 value and Alveolar–arterial (A–a) gradient, and in assessing if the alveoli are adequately transferring oxygen into the pulmonary circulation.

The equation assumes:
(1) inspired gas contains no CO_2 or water;
(2) the alveolar and arterial partial pressures of CO_2 are in equilibrium;
(3) the alveolar gas is saturated with water;
(4) the inspired and alveolar gases obey the ideal gas law.

RQ varies with diet (refer to page 136).

Clinical application/worked example

1. *A patient in the resuscitation bay, breathing 50% oxygen, has the following arterial blood gas results:*

$P_aO_2 = 14\,kPa$

$P_aCO_2 = 6.4\,kPa$

Calculate their Alveolar–arterial (A–a) gradient

We know that: $P_AO_2 = P_iO_2 - (P_ACO_2/RQ)$.

In calculating P_iO_2, we need to take into consideration water vapour pressure 6.3 kPa.

$(P_iO_2 = F_iO_2 \times (PATM - PH_2O))$

So: **$P_AO_2 = (0.5 \times (101 - 6.3)) - (6.4/0.8) = 39.4\,kPa.$**

Therefore: **A – a gradient = 39.4 – 14**

= 25.4 kPa.

2. *Why do anaesthetists prescribe oxygen in the immediate post-operative period?*

Post-operatively, patients often arrive in the recovery area hypoventilating. This may be due to a number of factors, including opiate administration, or the residual effects of anaesthetic agents. As a result, the patient's P_ACO_2 rises, which in turn, as demonstrated by the alveolar gas equation, causes their P_AO_2 to drop because they are reciprocal. To counteract this, supplementary oxygen is delivered to increase the P_iO_2 and subsequently, a greater P_AO_2.

Helium dilution technique

$$V_2 = V_1 \times \left(\frac{C_1 - C_2}{C_2} \right)$$

Definition of terms used

V_2 = total gas volume (functional residual capacity + spirometer volume)
V_1 = volume of gas in spirometer
C_1 = initial known helium concentration
C_2 = final helium concentration (measured by spirometer)

Units

Units of volume = litres.

Explanation

The helium dilution technique is a method of measuring the functional residual capacity (FRC) of the lungs (refer to page 128). A closed-circuit technique is used in which subjects are asked to inhale and exhale through a spirometer containing a known concentration of helium and oxygen. As helium is virtually insoluble in blood and thus not lost from the circuit, over time the helium concentrations in the lung and spirometer equilibrate, and consequently the volume of the FRC can be calculated (see derivation below).

In patients with obstructive lung disease, this method of measuring FRC may not be reliable due to incomplete equilibration of helium throughout the lung. In this instance another technique, body plethysmography, should be used.

Clinical application/worked example

1. *Calculate the FRC of a subject using the helium dilution method.*
   Spirometer helium concentration: 10%
   Spirometer volume: 5 litres
   Helium concentration after equilibration: 7%

Using the calculation above:

FRC = 5 × (10 − 7)/7

= 2.1 litres

Derivation

(1) *The spirometer contains a known volume of gas (V_1) with a known concentration of helium in it (C_1).*

(2) *Therefore, the amount of helium present in the spirometer before equilibrium*

$$= C_1 \times V_1$$

(3) *Once the patient starts breathing, the helium concentration will drop as it gets diluted within the patient's lungs and the spirometer. Therefore, the amount of helium present after equilibrium*

$$= C_2 \times (V_1 + V_2)$$

(4) *Thus*

$$V_2 (= FRC)$$

(5) V_1, C_1 and C_2 are all known values. Therefore:

$$V_2 = V_1 \times \left(\frac{C_1 - C_2}{C_2} \right)$$

Spirometry: forced expiration

$$Ratio = \frac{FEV_1}{FVC}$$

Definition of terms used

FEV_1 = forced expiratory volume in one second
FVC = forced vital capacity

Units

Nil – it is a ratio.

Normal = .80 (= 80%).

Explanation

This simple equation allows one to distinguish between restrictive and obstructive lung diseases.

In obstructive disease, for example asthma and chronic obstructive airways disease (COAD), while the FVC may be normal or mildly decreased, FEV_1 is far more reduced due to increased airway resistance to expiratory flow. This gives a low FEV_1/FVC, and typically values of < 80% are demonstrated.

In restrictive disease such as pulmonary fibrosis, the FVC and FEV_1 are both decreased, and consequently the FEV_1/FVC value will be normal or increased.

Clinical application/worked example

1. *A breathless patient in the clinic presents with the following spirometry results: $FEV_1 = 2.5\,l$, $FVC = 4\,l$. Suggest whether this is a normal, obstructive or restrictive picture.*

   From the equation above, 2.5/4 = 63%.
   Therefore, this is an obstructive picture, and may represent asthma or COAD.

Lung volumes and capacities

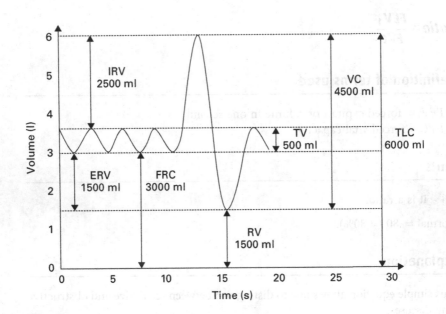

Definition of terms used

See below.

Units

ml.

Explanation

These refer to the volume of gas associated with different phases of the respiratory cycle. Importantly:
(1) lung volumes are discrete measurements of specific entities;
(2) lung capacities are two or more volumes added together.

As seen from the above diagram, there are multiple ways in which these can be calculated.

   (i) **Total Lung Capacity (TLC)** = Inspiratory Reserve Volume (IRV) + Tidal Volume (TV) + Expiratory Reserve Volume (ERV) + Residual Volume (RV).
   (ii) **Functional Residual Capacity (FRC)** = ERV + RV.
   (iii) **Vital Capacity (VC)** = IRV + TV + ERV.
   (iv) **Tidal Volume (TV)** = Alveolar Volume (V_A) + Anatomical dead space (V_d) (normal = 7 ml/kg).
   (v) **Inspiratory Capacity (IC)** = IRV + TV.
   (vi) **Expiratory Capacity** = TV + ERV.

(NB: TV interchangeable, elsewhere stated as V_t.)

Respiratory quotient and respiratory exchange ratio

$$RQ = VCO_2/VO_2$$

Definition of terms used

RQ = respiratory quotient
VCO_2 = carbon dioxide exhaled
VO_2 = oxygen uptake

Units

A quotient is, by its nature, dimensionless. The two gases must have the same units and in quantities proportional to the number of molecules (e.g. ml/kg/min). However, they cancel each other out to give RQ.

Explanation

The respiratory quotient (or respiratory coefficient) is used in the calculation of basal metabolic rate over a time period, when estimated from carbon dioxide production using indirect calorimetry. It is also used in the alveolar gas equation (refer to page 123).

The range of the RQ normally varies from 1.0 (pure carbohydrate oxidation) to 0.7 (pure fat oxidation). It may be below 0.7 with hypoventilation or prolonged fasting, or above 1.0 with hyperventilation. In a mixed diet a value of 0.8 is considered as normal.

It may also be described as the Respiratory Exchange Ratio (RER); however, this is the ratio between the amount of CO_2 exhaled and O_2 consumed in one breath.

Clinical application/worked example

1. When undergoing a strenuous cardiopulmonary exercise test, how would you expect your RQ to change?

At complete rest, one's VCO_2 and VO_2 will be similar to cellular carbon dioxide production and oxygen consumption (QCO_2 and QO_2, respectively). As one starts to exercise gently, hyperventilation will increase both oxygen consumption and carbon dioxide production, although if we say the metabolic source has not altered, it will still be in the same ratio.

At anaerobic threshold (lactate threshold), where anaerobic ATP synthesis supplements aerobic ATP synthesis, lactic acid is produced, excess CO_2 is exhaled, and consequently the RQ increases as CO_2 production exceeds oxygen uptake.

Shunt equation

$$\frac{Q_S}{Q_T} = \frac{C_cO_2 - C_aO_2}{C_cO_2 - C_vO_2}$$

Definition of terms used

Q_S = shunted blood flow (bypassing oxygenation in the lungs)
Q_T = total blood flow (= cardiac output)
C_cO_2 = oxygen content of end pulmonary capillary blood
C_aO_2 = oxygen content of arterial blood
C_vO_2 = oxygen content of mixed venous blood

Units

Nil – given as a fraction or percentage.

Normal < 5%.

Explanation

The shunt equation quantifies the extent that venous blood bypasses oxygenation in the pulmonary capillaries of the lung.

In normal health, blood from the bronchial veins (draining the lung parenchyma), and the Thebesian veins (draining cardiac muscle), represents a physiological shunt of approximately 5% of cardiac output. This shunted fraction of total pulmonary blood flow will increase as more blood flows through non-ventilated segments of lung whatever the underlying cause.

Hypoxia caused by shunted blood cannot be remedied by breathing 100% oxygen, as the shunted blood bypasses ventilated alveoli.

Clinical application/worked example

1. *Calculate the shunt for a patient who is found to have:*
   Mixed venous blood oxygen content of 15 ml O_2/dl,
   Pulmonary capillary oxygen content of 20 ml O_2/dl
   Systemic arterial blood oxygen content of 18 ml O_2/dl

Using the above equation: $Q_S/Q_T = (20 - 18)/(20 - 15)$

$= 40\%$

Derivation

(1) *Total pulmonary blood flow is made up of blood passing through the pulmonary capillaries (Q_c) and blood that has bypassed the pulmonary capillaries (Q_s)*

$Q_T = Q_S + Q_c$

(2) Q_c *can be calculated by subtracting the shunted blood (Q_S) from the total blood flow (Q_T).*

$Q_c = Q_T - Q_S$

(3) *If we add the oxygen content to the equation first equation, we get the oxygen content of Q_T.*

$Q_T \times C_aO_2 = Q_S \times C_vO_2 + ((Q_T \times C_cO_2) - (Q_S \times C_cO_2))$

(4) *Multiply out of brackets, and get Q_S and Q_T terms on the same side*

$Q_S \times (C_cO_2 - C_vO_2) = Q_T \times (C_cO_2 - C_aO_2)$

(5) *Divide by Q_T and ($C_cO_2 - C_vO_2$)*

$$\frac{Q_S}{Q_T} = \frac{C_cO_2 - C_aO_2}{C_cO_2 - C_vO_2}$$

Pulmonary vascular resistance

$$PVR = \left(\frac{PAP - PAWP}{CO} \right) \times 80$$

Definition of terms used

PVR = pulmonary vascular resistance
PAP = pulmonary artery pressure (mean)
$PAWP$ = pulmonary artery wedge pressure (mean)
CO = cardiac output

Units

dyn·s/cm^5 or mmHg·min/l.

(The latter of these are known as Wood units. They are used for ease of deriving pressure (mmHg) and cardiac output (l/min).)

Normal range 20–130 dyn·s/cm^5 or 0.25–1.6 Woods units.

Explanation

This equation defines the resistance attributable to the pulmonary flow, as opposed to the peripheral circulation (systemic vascular resistance or total peripheral resistance). The numerator describes the pressure difference between the input pressure (at the start of the pulmonary tree), and the output pressure (left atrium). In this calculation pulmonary artery wedge pressures have been described, however as this is an approximation of the left atrial pressure (LAP), this may be substituted and used instead.

The above equation also contains a numerical constant (80). This is to compensate for the units used if one wants to convert from mmHg·min/l to dyn·s/cm^5.

PVR can be indexed (PVRI) to body surface area (BSA) by substituting CO in the equation for cardiac index (CI). Normal range is 255–285 dyn·s/cm^5/m^2.

Clinical application/worked example

1. Estimate the pulmonary vascular resistance in this adult undergoing a liver resection.

$PAP = 15\,mmHg$

$LAP = 5\,mmHg$

$CO = 5\,l/min$

From the above equation: (15 − 5)/5

= 2 mmHg·min/l

2. What happens to the PVR at altitude?

At altitude, because of the diminished partial pressure of oxygen, hypoxic pulmonary vasoconstriction occurs in the lungs. Because of the uniform increased resistance occurring throughout the lung, in order to maintain a constant cardiac output, one's pulmonary artery pressure increases accordingly.

3. List some of the causes of pulmonary hypertension in patients in the intensive care unit.

  (i) Pre-existing pulmonary arterial hypertension (PAH).
 (ii) Elevated left atrial pressure (= PAWP), e.g. mitral regurgitation, cardiomyopathy, myocardial infarction.
(iii) Hypoxia, as explained above.
(iv) Thromboembolic, e.g. acute pulmonary embolism.
 (v) Iatrogenic, for example due to raised plateau pressures during mechanical ventilation.
(vi) Drugs, for example the use of norepinephrine or phosphodiesterase inhibitors.

Renal filtration fraction

$$FF = \frac{GFR}{RPF}$$

Definition of terms used

FF = filtration fraction
GFR = glomerular filtration rate
RPF = renal plasma flow

Units

Nil.

Explanation

The renal filtration fraction gives the proportion of plasma filtered at the glomeruli. Of the total renal blood flow (1 l/min), only the plasma (600 ml/min) has the potential to be filtered. In normal health, with a GFR of 125 ml/min, this approximates to 20%.

Clinical application/worked example

1. *Discuss situations in which the renal filtration fraction may change.*

Renal artery stenosis reduces renal blood flow, and thus in order to maintain the normal renal function, glomerular filtration rate increases and consequently renal filtration fraction increases.
Thiazide and loop diuretics decrease the filtration fraction.

Renal clearance and Cockcroft–Gault formula

$$Cx = \frac{Ux \times V}{Px}$$

Definition of terms used

Cx = renal clearance of x
Ux = urine concentration of x
V = urine flow
Px = plasma concentration of x

Units

ml/min.

Explanation

The clearance of any substance excreted by the kidney is the volume of plasma that is cleared of the substance per unit time. This is analogous to the clearance equation for any drug, UV/P (refer to page 55).

Clearance represents a theoretical volume of plasma cleared of the substance per unit time; however, physiologically, no quantity of plasma is completely cleared of a substance as it passes through the kidney.

Creatinine is routinely used clinically to assess clearance, and thus give an indication of renal function through an approximation of the glomerular filtration rate (GFR). It is freely filtered, not reabsorbed, synthesized or metabolized by the kidney and therefore its plasma levels remain relatively constant. However, the peritubular capillaries also actively secrete creatinine such that creatinine clearance overestimates actual GFR by 10–20%, and in practice, GFR is usually calculated using, for example, the Cockcroft–Gault formula (Donald Cockcroft, Henry Gault, 1976):

$$eC_{cr} = \frac{(140 - age) \times Mass \times K}{Creatinine_{serum}}$$

K = constant (1.23 in males, 1.04 in females)
Mass (kg)
Creatinine (µmol/l)

Clinical application/worked example

1. *Calculate the creatinine clearance (C_{Cr}) for the following patient in the intensive care unit:*

   24 hour urine volume = 1440 ml
   24 hour urine creatinine amount = 1440 mg
   Urine concentration = 1 mg/ml
   Plasma concentration = 0.01 mg/ml

$$C_{Cr} = (U_{Cr} \times V_{Cr})/P_{Cr}$$

$$= (1 \times 1440)/0.01$$

$$= 144{,}000 \text{ in 24 hours}$$

$$= 100 \text{ ml/min}$$

2. *Using the Cockcroft–Gault formula, calculate the estimated creatinine clearance for the following male patient:*

   Age 67
   Weight 89
   Serum creatinine 387

$$eC_{cr} = \frac{(140 - age) \times \text{Mass} \times K}{\text{Creatinine}_{serum}}$$

$$eC_{cr} = \frac{(140 - 67) \times 89 \times 1.23}{387}$$

$$= 20.6 \text{ ml/min}$$

Starling's equation – rate of filtration

$$Jv = k \times (P_c + \Pi_i) - (P_i + \Pi_c)$$

Definition of terms used

Jv = net fluid movement across capillary wall
k = filtration coefficient
P_c = hydrostatic pressure in the capillary
P_i = hydrostatic pressure in the interstitium
π_i = colloidal osmotic pressure in the interstitium
π_c = colloidal osmotic pressure in the capillary

Units

ml/min.

Explanation

The Starling equation (Ernest Starling, 1896) illustrates the role of hydrostatic and oncotic forces (the so-called Starling forces) in the movement of fluid across capillary membranes.

The first part of the equation describes the forces favouring filtration and the second half describes the forces opposing filtration. Therefore, net filtration is proportional to net driving force.

The filtration coefficient is the constant of proportionality. A high value indicates a highly water-permeable capillary, and vice versa.

Clinical application/worked example

1. Use Starling's equation to discuss the glomerular rate of filtration.

The forces governing glomerular filtration are the hydrostatic pressure gradients and the oncotic pressure gradients. These can be described as the forces favouring filtration (glomerular capillary hydrostatic pressure plus oncotic pressure in the

Bowman's capsule) minus the forces opposing filtration (hydrostatic pressure in the Bowman's capsule plus the oncotic pressure in the glomerular capillaries).

$$GFR \propto (P_{cap} - \Pi_{bc}) - (P_{bc} + \Pi_{cap})$$

(P_{cap} = hydrostatic pressure in capillary, Π_{bc} = oncotic pressure in Bowman's capsule, P_{bc} = hydrostatic pressure in Bowman's capsule, Π_{cap} = oncotic pressure in capillary.)

Normally, P_{cap} is 45 mmHg, P_{bc} is 10 mmHg, π_{bc} is zero as negligible amounts of protein enter the Bowman's capsule, and π_{cap} changes as filtration proceeds along the glomerulus.

The net fluid filtration per day in the glomerulus is about 125 ml/min or 180 l/day.

Fick's law of diffusion

$$Vgas \propto \left(\frac{A}{T}\right) \times D \times (P_1 - P_2)$$

And

$$D \propto \frac{Sol}{\sqrt{MW}}$$

Definition of terms used

$Vgas$ = volume of gas diffused
A = area
T = thickness
D = diffusion constant
$P_1 - P_2$ = difference in partial pressure (also described as ΔP)
Sol = gas solubility
MW = molecular weight

Units

ml/min.

Explanation

Fick's law (Adolf Fick, 1855) describes diffusion of a gas through tissues and can, if required, be used to solve the diffusion coefficient. In clinical terms, it is normally used to describe the movement of oxygen and carbon dioxide down a concentration gradient. Remember that diffusion is always a passive process that requires no energy.

The equation states that:

(1) the rate of diffusion of a gas through tissues is proportional to the:
- surface area (A),
- difference in gas partial pressure between the two sides (ΔP), and
- solubility of gas in the tissue (Sol); and

(2) the rate of diffusion is inversely proportional to the:
- thickness of the tissue (T), and
- the square root of the molecular weight of the gas (MW).

In other words, the larger the area, difference in concentration and the thinner the surface, the quicker the rate of diffusion.

The diffusion constant depends upon the properties of the tissue and gas in question, such that CO_2 diffuses about 20 times more readily than oxygen through the blood–gas barrier in the lungs.

Clinical application/worked example

1. *Describe the factors that may affect the diffusion of a gas across the blood–gas barrier.*

If the gas in question remained the same gas, then this would not alter factors relating to the diffusion constant (solubility and molecular weight). Altering factors would thus include the area and thickness of the blood–gas barrier (such as fibrosis), and difference in partial pressure of gas (such as alveolar hypoxia).

2. *Using Fick's Law, what features in the lung make diffusion more efficient?*

- The surface area (A) is very large due to the presence of millions of alveoli.
- The difference in partial pressure of the gases is maintained by breathing and pulmonary blood flow.
- The alveolar walls are only one cell thick (T).

Osmolality/osmolarity and the osmolar gap

Osmolality = (2 × Na) + Glucose + Urea

Osmolarity = (2 × Na) + Glucose + Urea

Definition of terms used

Osmolality = number of osmoles of solute per kilogram of solvent (mOsmol/kg)

Osmolarity = number of osmoles of solute per litre of solution (mOsmol/l)

Na = plasma sodium (mmol/l)

Glucose = plasma glucose (mmol/l)

Urea = plasma urea (mmol/l)

NB: Osmolality and osmolarity are technically different with dissimilar units of measurement. However, at low concentrations (below about 500 mOsmol), the mass of the solute is negligible compared to the mass of the solvent, and osmolarity and osmolality are very similar.

Units

Osmolality (mOsmol/kg).

Osmolarity (mOsmol/l).

The normal osmolality of extracellular fluid is 280–295 mOsmol/kg.

Explanation

Plasma osmolality or osmolarity is a measure of the osmolar concentration of plasma and is proportional to the number of particles per kilogram of solvent or litre of solution, respectively. In general, osmolality is a measured value using an osmometer and osmolarity is derived using the equation.

It is derived from the measured sodium, urea and glucose concentrations, which under normal circumstances contribute nearly all of the osmolality of the sample. The doubling of the sodium accounts for the negative ions associated with sodium, and the exclusion of potassium approximates for the incomplete dissociation of sodium chloride.

The osmolar (osmotic) gap (OG), is an indiscriminate measure of the difference between the actual laboratory measured osmolality (using an osmometer), and the calculated osmolarity.

Normally this value is $< 10\,mOsmol/kg$; however, it may be increased in situations depending on the presence of other osmotically active solutes which are measured but not taken into account in your calculation. It does not identify these abnormal solutes but rather alerts you to their presence.

Causes of raised OG include methanol, ethanol and ethylene glycol ingestion.

Clinical application/worked example

1. *Calculate the osmolar gap for this patient presenting in the Emergency Department with a decreased level of consciousness, and describe the result.*

Hb	10.4 g/dl
Na	134 mmol/l
K	3.7 mmol/l
HCO₃	23 mmol/l
Urea	4.4 mmol/l
Creatinine	74 mmol/l
Glucose	12.1 mmol/l
Serum osmolality	324 mOsm/l

Calculated serum osmolarity: $(2 \times 134) + 12.1 + 4.4 = 284.5$

Calculated osmolar gap: $324 - 284.5 = 39.5$

This is a markedly elevated osmolar gap, and suggests the presence of other osmotically active solutes, such as methanol, or ethylene glycol has been ingested, causing the clinical picture.

Morse equation and osmotic pressure

$$\Pi = iRTM$$

Definition of terms used

Π = osmotic pressure
R = universal gas constant
T = absolute temperature
M = molar concentration in mol/l
i = van't Hoff factor (empirical constant related to the degree of dissociation of the solute).

Units

Unit of pressure, e.g. atm.

Explanation

Osmotic pressure is the hydrostatic pressure that needs to be applied to a solution to prevent the inward flow of water across a semipermeable membrane. An osmotic imbalance between cells and their surroundings, such as with the administration of hypotonic fluid, may cause cytolysis (cell bursting due to excess intracellular water).

This is therefore vital in cell biology, as solvents, mainly water, will move across semipermeable membranes, from areas of low concentration to areas of high concentration, by osmosis. This will increase the pressure of the compartment, and the pressure required to oppose the movement of water is known as the osmotic pressure.

The osmotic pressure of an ideal solution may be estimated using the Morse equation (Harmon Morse, 1914). The equation is based on the van't Hoff equation (Jacobus van't Hoff, 1887) relating to chemical thermodynamics. It is remarkably similar to the universal gas equation (refer to page 9), which relates to the fact that dilute solutions behave in a similar way to gases.

Clinical application/worked example

1. Explain the importance of osmotic pressure when administering intravenous fluids to a critically ill patient.

When isotonic fluids are administered, water movement in and out of the cells is negligible. However, when hypotonic solutions such as 0.45% sodium chloride are given, water will move in to the cells until the osmotic pressure within the cell opposes any further movement. However, this may result in cell lysis, which is especially important in those patients with brain injuries.

Conversely, hypertonic solutions will encourage fluid out of the intracellular and interstitial spaces in to the intravascular compartment until the osmotic pressure opposes this. This may be beneficial in some cases, for example to reduce cerebral oedema, but can cause circulatory overload and cardiac failure in susceptible patients.

2. How do plasma proteins contribute to the osmotic pressure?

In normal plasma, the plasma proteins are the major colloids present (particles of large molecular weight). Because the colloids are solutes, they contribute to the total osmotic pressure. This component is referred to as the **colloid osmotic pressure** or **oncotic pressure**.

3. Use the van't Hoff equation to calculate the osmotic pressure for this typical plasma sample:

$T = 310K \ (= 37\,^{\circ}C)$

$R = 0.082 \ l{\cdot}atm/mol{\cdot}K$

$i = 1$ *(because plasma proteins do not dissociate)*

$M = 0.280 \ mol/l$

Using the equation, $\Pi = iRTM$

$\Pi = 1 \times 0.082 \times 310 \times 0.280$

$\Pi = 7.12$ atm.

Anion gap

Anion gap = ([Na$^+$] + [K$^+$]) − ([Cl$^-$] + [HCO$_3^-$])

Definition of terms used

Cations:
    [Na$^+$] = concentration of sodium ions
    [K$^+$] = concentration of potassium ions
Anions:
    [Cl$^-$] = concentration of chloride ions
    [HCO$_3^-$] = concentration of bicarbonate ions

(NB: *[K$^+$] may be omitted in some formulae as its concentration is relatively low compared to the other three ions and typically does not change much.)

Units

Concentrations are expressed in units of milliequivalents/litre (mEq/l) or in millimoles/litre (mmol/l).

Normal = 8–16 mmol/l or 10–20 mEq/l (although this varies between sources).

Explanation

The anion gap is a calculated measure that is representative of the unmeasured anions in serum (and urine). It usually uses cations ([Na$^+$] + [K$^+$]) and anions ([Cl$^-$] + [HCO$_3^-$]) for its calculation, and the magnitude of this difference or gap allows identification of the cause of a metabolic acidosis. This is because the acid anions such as lactate, acetoacetate or sulphate are not always routinely measured. It may be classed as either high, normal or, in rare cases, low.

In normal health there are more measurable cations compared to measurable anions in the serum and therefore the anion gap is usually positive. The negatively charged proteins account for the majority of the normal anion gap. Because we know that plasma is electro-neutral we can conclude that the anion gap calculation represents the concentration of unmeasured anions.

Clinical application/worked example

1. Describe a pathological situation which may result in an altered anion gap.

The anion gap can be classified as high, normal or low.

A high anion gap indicates a metabolic acidosis such as that encountered in diabetic ketoacidosis. In an attempt to buffer the unmeasured H^+ cations, bicarbonate concentrations decrease, thereby resulting in a high anion gap.

Other causes of a raised anion gap could be: methanol, uraemia, diabetic ketoacidosis, salicylate overdose and lactic acidosis.

A normal anion gap acidosis is a hyperchloraemic acidosis due to loss of HCO_3^-.

A low anion gap is found in hypoalbuminaemia, for example cirrhosis, haemorrhage and nephrotic syndrome.

Note that the anion gap decreases by 2.5–3 mmol/l for every 1 g decrease in albumin.

Goldman equation

$$Em = \left(\frac{RT}{F}\right) \times \ln \frac{P_k[K^+]_o + P_{Na}[Na^+]_o + P_{Cl}[Cl^-]_o}{P_k[K^+]_i + P_{Na}[Na^+]_i + P_{Cl}[Cl^-]_i}$$

Definition of terms used

Em = membrane potential
P_i = membrane permeability for the ion in question (Na, K, Cl)
$[ion]_i$ = intracellular concentration of the ion
$[ion]_o$ = extracellular concentration of the ion
R = universal gas constant
T = temperature
F = Faraday's constant

Units

mV.

Explanation

The Goldman equation is otherwise known as the Goldman constant field equation, or the Goldman–Hodgkin–Katz equation (David Goldman, Alan Hodgkin, Bernard Katz).

While the Nernst equation (refer to page 153) provides a quantitative measure of the equality that exists between chemical and electrical gradients for individual ions, the Goldman equation calculates the predicted resting membrane potential (RMP) that reflects the relative contributions of the chemical concentration gradients and relative membrane permeability for a multitude of ions collectively.

Usually these ions are potassium, sodium and chloride ions – the major contributors to the membrane potential.

The RMP of each cell is generated by the semipermeable nature of cell membranes and is key to understanding the movement of ions into and out of the cell. The importance of this equation, or rather what it represents, is difficult to over-emphasize, as the presence of the transmembrane electrical differences is the basis for all cellular function.

Clinical application/worked example

1. What are the resting membrane potentials for the following cell types?

Skeletal muscle cells
Smooth muscle cells
Astroglia
Neurons
Cardiac myocyte
Cardiac pacemaker cell

Answer

Skeletal muscle cells	−95 mV
Smooth muscle cells	−60 mV
Astroglia	−80 to −90 mV
Neurons	−60 to −70 mV
Cardiac myocyte	−90 mV
Cardiac pacemaker cell	−60 mV

Gibbs–Donnan effect

Anion A × Cation A = Anion B × Cation B

Definition of terms used

Anion A = number of permeable anions on side A
Cation A = number of permeable cations on side A
Anion B = number of permeable anions on side B
Cation B = number of permeable cations on side B

Units

Nil.

Explanation

The Gibbs–Donnan effect (Josiah Gibbs, Frederick Donnan, 1911) describes the behaviour of charged particles across a semipermeable membrane. Because some particles cannot diffuse across the membrane (e.g. proteins), their electrostatic presence will result in the asymmetric distribution of permeable ions. In vivo, this mainly results in the movement of sodium and chloride ions between the intravascular and interstitial body compartments.

Ultimately, as described in the equation, the diffusible anions and cations are distributed across the two sides of the membrane so that:
(1) the products of their concentrations are equal, and
(2) the sum of the permeable and impermeable anions on either side is equal to that of the permeable and impermeable cations on either side.
This ultimately achieves electro-neutrality across both sides of the membrane.

The balance between the chemical and electrostatic forces produces an electrical potential difference that can be calculated using the Nernst equation (refer to page 153).

Clinical application/worked example

1. Where is the Gibbs–Donnan effect demonstrable in the intensive care unit?

Critically ill patients requiring renal replacement therapy are often prescribed haemodialysis. Here, the dialysis solution is carefully regulated to dictate the movement of ions between the plasma and the dialysate.

Sodium movement is principally regulated by the ionic activity rather than the total sodium concentration. Plasma proteins are negatively charged and not diffusible through the dialysis membrane thereby setting up an electrostatic gradient across the membrane. The Gibbs–Donnan effect dictates that sodium, as the principle cation, will cross the membrane into the plasma to restore electrochemical neutrality.

Nernst equation

$$E = \left(\frac{RT}{zF}\right) \times \ln\left(\frac{[C]_o}{[C]_i}\right)$$

Definition of terms used

E = equilibrium potential
R = universal gas constant
T = temperature
z = valency (the number of valence bonds a given atom can form with one or more other atoms)
F = Faraday's constant
$[C]_o$ = concentration of ion outside the cell
$[C]_i$ = concentration of ion inside the cell

Units

mV.

Explanation

The Nernst equation (Walther Nernst, 1864–1941) provides a formula that relates the numerical values of the concentration gradient to the electrical gradient that balances it.

The equation is used to calculate the potential difference that any individual ion would produce if the membrane were fully permeable to it. Therefore, it is able to give a value for the voltage that must exist across a membrane in order to balance a chemical gradient that exists for the ion in question.

However, at rest, the cell membrane is more permeable to some ions than others (semipermeable). This creates an equilibrium whereby the electrical forces pulling an ion in to or out of a cell are exactly opposed by the concentration gradient pulling the ion in the opposite direction. If the concentration difference for a given ion across the membrane is known ($[C]_o/[C]_i$), then the equilibrium potential can be calculated using the Nernst equation.

In practice, we can take R, T, and F to be constant and z is determined by the electrical charge of ion in question. Therefore, the larger the discrepancy, the greater the Nernst potential required to prevent diffusion.

Clinical application/worked example

1. Describe the Nernst potential for potassium and sodium in a cell in its resting state.

At rest, excitable cell membranes such as those found in cardiac myocytes are nearly fully permeable to potassium (K^+). Therefore, the equilibrium potential for K^+ is comparable to the cell's resting membrane potential (RMP) of approximately –90 mV.

Because of this, changes in the extracellular potassium concentration can have a profound effect on the RMP. In cardiac myocytes, an elevated serum potassium concentration can markedly increase the likelihood of the cell depolarizing, thereby increasing the risk of arrhythmias.

As the same cell membranes are comparatively impermeable to sodium (Na^+), this ion has an equilibrium potential of approximately +80 mV. As Na^+ movement across the cell membrane is much more dependent on ion channels, a change in the extracellular concentration is much less likely to cause clinical symptoms. This is manifest in the fact that the 'normal range' of Na^+ in clinical practice is 4–5 times as large as that of K^+.

pH

pH = − log[H⁺]

pH = $-\log[H^+]$

Definition of terms used

[H⁺] = hydrogen ion concentration in a given solution.

$[H^+]$ = hydrogen ion concentration in a given solution.

Units

The pH has an arbitrary scale of 1 to 14.
$[H^+]$ concentration is measured in nmol/l.

Explanation

pH (Søren Sorensen, 1909), quoted as the 'negative logarithm of the hydrogen ion concentration $[H^+]$', represents the activity of hydrogen ions within a given solution. (The meaning of 'p' is unclear, but probably refers to 'power'.)

As the equation uses a negative logarithm, for each reduction by one in pH, there is a 10-fold increase in $[H^+]$ activity. For example, a 0.1 unit fall in pH from 7.4 to 7.3 represents a 25% increase in $[H^+]$ activity.

The pH of pure water is about 7 at 25 °C; acids have a pH lower than this, and alkaline solutions have a pH higher than this. Most measured values lie in the range from 0 to 14. However, within the body, the pH of various body compartments is tightly regulated through homeostatic mechanisms. The normal range for blood is 7.34–7.45, whereas gastric acid has a pH around 1.

Clinical application/worked example

Calculate the [H$^+$] concentrations in nM/dl for the following pH values.

pH
5.00
6.00
7.00
7.40
8.00
9.00

Answer

pH	[H$^+$] (nM/dl)
5.00	10,000
6.00	1,000
7.00	100
7.40	40
8.00	10
9.00	1

pKa

pKa = − logKa

Definition of terms used

Ka = acid dissociation constant
(NB: this may be written as K_d.)

Units

Nil.

Explanation

pKa represents the negative logarithmic measure of the acid dissociation constant (Ka). The acid dissociation constant is the equilibrium constant for the dissociation of acid–base reactions and gives a quantitative measure of the strength of an acid in a solution.

A given generic acid (HA) will dissociate into its conjugate base (A^-) and hydrogen ions or proton [H^+]. The chemical species are said to be in equilibrium when their concentrations do not change with the passing of time:

$$HA \Leftrightarrow A^- + H^+$$

The dissociation constant is usually written as a quotient of the equilibrium concentrations (in mol/l)

$$Ka = \frac{[A^-][H^+]}{[HA]}$$

The lower the pKa, the higher the extent of dissociation and thus pH of the solution.

The concept of pKa is important to understand in relation to membrane permeability within the body. Most drugs exist as either weak acids or weak bases and therefore in ionized and unionized forms depending on the pH of the environment. In general, only the unionized form can cross the cell membrane.

For a drug that is a WEAK BASE (e.g. local anaesthetics):

$BH = B^- + H^+$

the dissociation constant is given by the Henderson–Hasselbalch equation (refer to page 161):

$pKa = pH + \log[BH]/[B^-]$

In an acidic environment, the equation will tend towards the left (the ionized form) and in an alkaline environment, the equation will tend towards the right (the unionized form).

For a drug that is a WEAK ACID (e.g. aspirin):

$AH = A^- + H^+$

the dissociation constant is given by the Henderson–Hasselbalch equation (refer to page 161):

$pKa = pH + \log[AH]/[A^-]$

In an acidic environment, the equation will tend towards the left (the unionized form) and in an alkaline environment, the equation will tend towards the right (the ionized form). This is opposite to the weak bases.

Clinical application/worked example

1. Describe the importance of pKa and local anaesthetics.

Local anaesthetics are weak bases, such that they exist in ionized (BH^+) and unionized (B) forms. Their pKa defines the pH at which equilibrium is reached between the two forms, and also determines the amount of local anaesthetic in each form at any given pH.

At the physiological pH of 7.4, 25% of lignocaine (pKa 7.9) is in the unionized form, and 15% of bupivacaine (pKa 8.1). It is this unionized form that is important in determining the speed of onset for local anaesthetics, as this is the form that crosses the nerve cell membrane.

This explains why the drug with the lower pKa (lignocaine), and consequently more unionized in nature, will reach the target site and act more quickly.

2. Why is aspirin well absorbed from the stomach?

Aspirin is a weak acid and so in the highly acidic environment of the stomach, more of the unionized form exists, which enables the drug to cross the cell membrane.

Acid–base compensation simplified

$$\text{pH} \propto HCO_3^- / P_a CO_2$$

Definition of terms used

pH = negative logarithm of the hydrogen ion concentration $[H^+]$
HCO_3^- = concentration of bicarbonate in blood
$P_a CO_2$ = partial pressure of CO_2 in blood

Units

Nil.

Explanation

This simplified version of the Henderson–Hasselbalch equation disregards the pK and log, and describes the relationship among the three fundamental values. It allows for easy description of acid–base disturbances and their compensatory changes.

Clinical application/worked example

(1) Respiratory acidosis: $\uparrow P_a CO_2$

Principle event: $\downarrow\text{pH} = HCO_3^- / \uparrow P_a CO_2$

Metabolic compensation: $\text{pH} = \uparrow HCO_3^- / P_a CO_2$

(2) Respiratory alkalosis: $\downarrow P_a CO_2$

Principle event: $\uparrow\text{pH} = HCO_3^- / \downarrow P_a CO_2$

Metabolic compensation: $\text{pH} = \downarrow HCO_3^- / P_a CO_2$

(3) Metabolic alkalosis: $\uparrow HCO_3^-$

Principle event: $\uparrow$pH = $\uparrow HCO_3^- / P_a CO_2$

Metabolic compensation: pH = $HCO_3^- / \uparrow P_a CO_2$

(4) Metabolic acidosis: $\downarrow HCO_3^-$

Principle event: $\downarrow$pH = $\downarrow HCO_3^- / P_a CO_2$

Metabolic compensation: pH = $HCO_3^- / \downarrow P_a CO_2$.

Henderson–Hasselbalch equation

$$pH = pKa + \log \frac{[A^-]}{[HA]}$$

Modified version to relate the pH of blood to constituents of the bicarbonate buffering system.

$$pH = pKa + \log \left(\frac{[HCO_3^-]}{[H_2CO_3]} \right)$$

Or

$$pH = \frac{[HCO_3^-]}{P_aCO_2}$$

Definition of terms used

pH = negative logarithm of the hydrogen ion concentration $[H^+]$ (refer to page 155)

pKa = negative logarithmic measure of the acid dissociation constant (Ka) (refer to page 157)

$[HCO_3^-]$ = concentration of bicarbonate in blood

$[H_2CO_3]$ = concentration of carbonic acid in blood

P_aCO_2 = partial pressure of CO_2 in blood

Units

Arbitrary logarithmic scale from 0 to 14.

Explanation

The Henderson–Hasselbalch equation (Lawrence Joseph Henderson and Karl Albert Hasselbalch, 1908) describes the derivation of pH as a measure of acidity in biological and chemical systems. We often encounter it in clinical practice when referring to acid–base homeostasis to maintain a constant plasma pH.

Of the many buffer systems, the bicarbonate buffer system is quantitatively the largest, and most important, in extracellular fluid, and reflects any acid–base disturbances in either of its buffer components. In this system carbon dioxide

(CO_2) combines with water to form carbonic acid (H_2CO_3), which in turn rapidly dissociates to hydrogen ions [H^+] and bicarbonate (HCO_3^-).

$$H_2O + CO_2 \leftrightarrow H_2CO_3 \leftrightarrow H^+ + HCO_3^-$$

Clinical application/worked example

1. How do the equations help to explain acid–base homeostasis?

The equations are key to understanding the body's compensation to acid–base abnormalities. CO_2 and HCO_3^- are the two main variables that can be altered. According to the law of mass action, each side of the equation must remain balanced. Therefore, a rise in $PaCO_2$ in the blood (a respiratory acidosis) will shift the equation towards the right and cause a rise in bicarbonate in order to regain a normal pH.

Equally, a drop in bicarbonate (a metabolic acidosis) will shift the equation towards the left and cause a drop in pCO_2 via a respiratory compensation.

Derivation using bicarbonate buffer system

pH = negative logarithmic value of the hydrogen ion concentration = $-\log$ [H^+]
pKa = acid dissociation constant = $-\log K_d$

(1) Bicarbonate buffer system

$$H_2O + CO_2 \leftrightarrow H_2CO_3 \leftrightarrow H^+ + HCO_3^-$$

(2) Formulate the dissociation constant (K_d) for the above equation.

$$K_d = [H^+][HCO_3^-]/[H_2CO_3]$$

(3) Take the log for each value

$$\log K_d = \log[H^+] + \log ([HCO_3^-]/[H_2CO_3])$$

(4) Rearrange 'log[H^+]'

$$\log K_d - \log[H^+] = \log ([HCO_3^-]/[H_2CO_3])$$

(5) Rearrange 'log K_d'

$$\underset{(pH)}{- \log [H+]} = \underset{(pKa)}{- \log K_d} + \log ([HCO_3^-]/[H_2CO_3])$$

(6) Rename as per the definitions above

$$pH = pKa + \log ([HCO_3^-]/[H_2CO_3]).$$

Cerebral perfusion pressure and intracranial pressure

CPP = MAP - ICP

Definition of terms used

CPP = cerebral perfusion pressure
MAP = mean arterial pressure
ICP = intracranial pressure

Units

mmHg.

Normal CPP: 70–80 (range 50–150) mmHg.
Normal ICP: 5–15 mmHg.

Explanation

Cerebral perfusion pressure is dependent on the pressure gradient between the inflowing arteries (MAP) and outflowing veins. Cerebral venous pressure is difficult to measure and thus taken as intracranial pressure (ICP), which can be measured directly using an intraparenchymal or intraventricular pressure transducer. On the occasion where central venous pressure (CVP) exceeds ICP, then CVP should be substituted for ICP in the equation.

Due to the high cerebral metabolic rate of oxygen consumption ($CMRO_2$ = 50 ml/min) cerebral blood flow (mean 50 ml/100 g/min) should be maintained over a range of systemic pressures. This is achieved through autoregulation through a poorly understood local vascular mechanism.

The pressure–volume relationship between ICP and intracranial volume is known as the Monro–Kellie hypothesis (or doctrine). It states: (1) intracranial volume can be determined from the sum of its contents: blood, CSF and tissue, and (2) as the intracranial compartment is incompressible and thus of fixed volume, any increase in volume of one of the cranial constituents must be compensated for by a decrease in volume of another.

Clinical application/worked example

1. How does the Cushing reflex relate to CPP?

The Cushing reflex (Harvey Cushing, 1869–1939) is comprised of the Cushing triad: hypertension, bradycardia and irregular Cheyne–Stokes' breathing. It is a sign of critically increased ICP.

From the above equation we can see that as ICP increases (for whatever cause), in order to maintain an appropriate cerebral perfusion pressure, MAP must also increase. Through peripheral vasoconstriction systemic blood pressure increases, and thus the CPP is maintained. The systemic hypertension is sensed locally by carotid artery baroreceptors, and in response, a vagal-induced bradycardia occurs.

2. How can knowledge of the CPP equation guide the management of a patient with traumatic brain injury?

Following a head injury, cerebral blood flow is often decreased due to the effects of raised ICP secondary to bleeding, the loss of normal autoregulation, and hypovolaemia secondary to other injuries in the multiple-injured patient. In order to prevent neuronal injury and secondary brain injury, the CPP must be maintained above 70 mmHg.

The equation dictates that MAP should be appropriately maintained and ICP controlled.

Intraocular pressure

$$IOP = \frac{F}{C} + PV$$

Definition of terms used

IOP = intraocular pressure
F = aqueous humour formation rate
C = aqueous humour outflow rate
PV = episcleral venous pressure

Units

mmHg.

Normal = 10–20 mmHg.

Explanation

Intraocular pressure, measured by a tonometer, is predominantly determined by the inflow (ciliary body) and outflow (trabecular meshwork and canal of Schlemm) of aqueous humour. The volume of vitreous humour in the posterior chamber of the eye changes according to the IOP; however, this takes 15–30 min to occur.

In a similar manner to intracranial pressure (refer to page 163), the orbital globe is a non-compliant sphere within a rigid box. Therefore, IOP can be affected by a change in the components within the orbit, or by external pressure.

PV is predominantly influenced by the central venous pressure (CVP). There-fore, in patients with glaucoma, it is important to avoid venous congestion.

Clinical application/worked example

1. Name some pharmacological examples that can alter intraocular pressure.

(i) Prostaglandin analogues (latanoprost, bimatoprost): these increase aqueous humour outflow.
(ii) Beta blockers (timolol): these decrease aqueous humour production.
(iii) Suxamethonium chloride: this temporarily increases intraocular pressure.
(iv) Pilocarpine: constricts the pupil to relieve acute angle glaucoma to reduce IOP.

2. How does prone positioning affect the IOP?

There are a number of ways that the eye can be affected when positioning a patient in the prone position, all of which can cause catastrophic post-operative blindness. These include inadvertent external pressure on the eye which may cause the IOP to rise, venous engorgement which raises the CVP and PV, or ischaemic optic neuropathy caused by hypotension.

Binary classification tests and 2 × 2 tables

Binary classification involves classifying members of a population into two groups depending on whether or not they have a property. In the medical context, this refers to determining if a patient has or has not got a disease, and the classification is based on the presence or absence of said disease.

Comparing these classifications with those achieved by a gold standard test allows us to evaluate a diagnostic test, such as a screening test or assay, and statistical methods such as sensitivity, specificity, positive predictive value and negative predictive value may be used. The notation is shown in the table below:

Test outcome	Condition present (as determined by gold standard testing)		
		Present (true)	Not present (false)
	Positive	True positive (TP)	False positive (FP)
	Negative	False negative (FN)	True negative (TN)

To compare the occurrence of a binary outcome variable between two exposure (or treatment) groups, the data can be displayed in a 2 × 2 table. This shows the frequency of individuals in the sample classified according to whether they experienced the disease outcome (or event), and according to whether they were exposed (or treated). The notation is shown in the table below:

Exposure	Outcome	
	Experienced disease	Did not experience disease
Exposed	a	b
Unexposed	c	d

Negative predictive value

$$NPV = \frac{TN}{(TN + FN)}$$

Definition of terms used

NPV = negative predictive value
TN = true negative
FN = false negative

Units

Percentage.

Explanation

The negative predictive value of a test allows one to ask of a clinical test: 'if the test result is negative, what is the likelihood that this patient does not have the disease?' It is the probability that a patient truly does not have the condition if a test is negative.

NPV, like PPV (positive predictive value) (refer to page 170), depends on the prevalence of the disease in the population, as well as on the sensitivity and specificity of the procedure used. Lowering the prevalence of true positives (TPs) lowers the PPV. Increasing the prevalence will decrease the NPV.

Clinical application/worked example

1. *Calculate the negative predictive value of this new test for serum* Legionella *antigens.*

New test outcome	*Legionella* antigens present (as determined by gold standard testing)	
	Present	Not present
Positive	*32*	*7*
Negative	*5 (FN)*	*131 (TN)*

$$NPV = \frac{TN}{(TN + FN)}$$

$$NPV = 131/(131 + 5)$$

$$= 96\%$$

Positive predictive value

$$PPV = \frac{TP}{(TP + FP)}$$

Definition of terms used

PPV = positive predictive value
TP = true positive
FP = false positive

Units

Percentage.

Explanation

The positive predictive value of a test allows one to ask of a clinical test: 'if the test result is positive, what is the likelihood that this patient has the disease?' It is the probability that a patient is truly positive if a test is positive.

PPV and NPV (negative predictive value) (refer to page 168) depend on the prevalence of the disease in the population, as well as on the sensitivity and specificity of the procedure used. Lowering the prevalence of TPs lowers the PPV. Increasing the prevalence will decrease the NPV.

Clinical application/worked example

1. *Calculate the positive predictive value of this new test for serum* Legionella *antigens.*

Test outcome	Legionella antigens present (as determined by gold standard testing)	
	Present	Not present
Positive	32 (TP)	7 (FP)
Negative	5	131

$$PPV = \frac{TP}{(TP + FP)}$$

$PPV = 32/(32 + 7)$

$= 82\%$

Specificity

$$Specificity = \frac{TN}{(TN + FP)}$$

Definition of terms used

TN = true negative
FP = false positive

Units

Percentage.

Explanation

Specificity describes a clinical test's ability to correctly identify patients who have *not* got the disease. It is the proportion of true negatives correctly identified as such.

If a test has a specificity of 75%, of those who do not have the disease, 75% will correctly test negative (true negative), and 25% will be identified as having the disease in its absence (false positive).

Ideally, a test needs to be both highly specific and sensitive (refer to page 174). If a clinical test is highly sensitive but not very specific, many people will be incorrectly identified as having the disease, when actually they do not.

Clinical application/worked example

1. *Calculate the specificity for a new exhaled breath analyzer used to screen for the presence of lung cancer.*

Test outcome	Lung cancer present (as determined by gold standard testing)	
	Present	Not present
Positive	*34*	*24 (FP)*
Negative	*12*	*30 (TN)*

$$Specificity = \frac{TN}{(TN + FP)}$$

Specificity = 30 / (30 + 24)

= 56%

Sensitivity

$$Sensitivity = \frac{TP}{(TP + FN)}$$

Definition of terms used

TP = true positive
FN = false negative

Units

Percentage.

Explanation

Sensitivity measures the ability of a clinical test to correctly identify those patients with the disease. In other words, it measures how sensitive the test is to picking up the disease's presence. It is the proportion of true positives correctly identified as such.

An optimal screening test will have both a high sensitivity and specificity (refer to page 172). However, there is an inverse relationship between the two measures: improving one will decrease the other.

If a test has a sensitivity of 75%, of those whom have the disease, 75% will test positive (true positive), and 25% will not be identified when they should test positive (false negatives), i.e. they will be unidentified cases.

Clinical application/worked example

1. *A new exhaled breath analyzer is used to screen for the presence of lung cancer. Calculate the sensitivity of the test.*

Test outcome	Lung cancer present (as determined by gold standard testing)	
	Present	Not present
Positive	32 (TP)	7
Negative	5 (FN)	131

$$Sensitivity = \frac{TP}{(TP + FN)}$$

Sensitivity = 32 / (32 + 5)

= 86%

Relative risk

$$RR = \frac{(a/(a+b))}{(c/(c+d))}$$

Or

$$RR = \frac{I_T}{I_C}$$

Definition of terms used

RR = relative risk (also known as a risk ratio)
a, b, c, d = see 2 × 2 table below in example
I_T = cumulative incidence in exposed (treatment) group
I_C = cumulative incidence in unexposed (control) group

Units

Nil.

Explanation

Relative risk describes the occurrence of an outcome event experienced by different exposure groups. It is a relative measure, and is used to measure the strength of an association between exposure and disease. It is calculated from the risk of an outcome event in the exposed group divided by the risk of an event in the unexposed group.

RR = risk when exposed / risk when not exposed

If RR = 1, there is no difference between the groups.
If RR = 0.5, exposure halves the risk of the outcome event.
If RR = 0.75, exposure reduces the risk of the outcome event by 25%.
If RR = 2, exposure doubles the risk of the outcome event.

Clinical application/worked example

1. From the 2 × 2 table, calculate the relative risk of cancer associated with smoking.

Exposure	Outcome	
	Lung cancer	No lung cancer
Smoker	*28 (a)*	*72 (b)*
Non-smoker	*4 (c)*	*96 (d)*

$$RR = \frac{(a/(a+b))}{(c/(c+d))}$$

$$RR = \frac{(28/(28+72)}{(4/(4+96)}$$

$$= 7$$

You are seven times more likely to get lung cancer if you smoke.

Relative risk reduction

$$RRR = \frac{ARR}{I_c}$$

Definition of terms used

RRR = relative risk reduction
ARR = absolute risk reduction
I_C = cumulative incidence in unexposed (control) group

Units

Percentage.

Explanation

The relative risk reduction, calculated by dividing the absolute risk reduction (ARR) by the control incidence, is the proportion by which the intervention reduces the event rate. It can be more useful than ARR, as it not only accounts for the effectiveness of a drug or treatment, but also for the relative chance of an incident occurring in the absence of treatment.

Clinical application/worked example

1. *100 hypertensive men were given a new anti-hypertensive drug, and 100 hypertensive men were given a placebo. The results were as below.*

Exposure	Outcome	
	BP improved	BP not improved
Given anti-hypertensive	*80*	*20*
Placebo	*60*	*40*

ARR = 20% (refer to page 180)

Calculate the RRR for this new drug.

$$RRR = \frac{ARR}{I_c}$$

RRR = 20/40 = .5

RRR = 50%

The incidence of hypertension was reduced from 40% with placebo to 20% with treatment, i.e. by half.

Absolute risk reduction

$$ARR = I_T - I_C$$

Definition of terms used

ARR = absolute risk reduction
I_T = cumulative incidence in exposed (treatment) group
I_C = cumulative incidence in unexposed (control) group

Units

Percentage.

The equation above gives an absolute number, but can also be converted to percentage.

Explanation

The absolute risk reduction is the difference in risk between the exposed group and the unexposed group. ARR measures the impact of exposure.

Clinical application/worked example

1. *100 hypertensive men were given a new anti-hypertensive drug, and 100 hypertensive men given a placebo. The results were as below.*

Exposure	Outcome	
	BP improved	BP not improved
Given anti-hypertensive	80	20
Placebo	60	40

Calculate the ARR for this new drug.

$$ARR = I_T - I_C$$
$$ARR = 80/100 - 60/100$$
$$= 0.8 - 0.6$$
$$= 0.2 = 20\%$$

Accuracy of test

$$Accuracy = \frac{(TP + TN)}{Total}$$

Definition of terms used

TP = true positive
TN = true negative
Total = total number

Units

Nil.

Explanation

Accuracy is a statistical measure of how well a test correctly identifies or excludes a condition. The tests in question are binary classification tests.

It is calculated from the proportion of true results (true positives and true negatives) to the total number of results.

Clinical application/worked example

1. *A new assay has been used to screen for* Clostridium difficile *in patients' blood samples. The results for 100 patients are as follows.*

Test outcome	Condition present (as determined by gold standard testing)	
	Present (true)	Not present (false)
Positive	34 (TP)	24
Negative	12	30 (TN)

Please calculate the accuracy of the test.

$$Accuracy = \frac{(TP + TN)}{Total}$$

Accuracy = (34 + 30)/100

= 64%

This is not a very accurate test.

Chi-squared test

$$\chi^2 = \Sigma \frac{(o - e)^2}{e}$$

Definition of terms used

χ^2 = Chi-squared
Σ = sum of
o = observed number
e = expected number

Units

Nil.

Explanation

The Chi-squared test is a statistical hypothesis test used for comparing the observed numbers in each cell of a 2 × 2 table with those we would expect if there was no relationship between the two variables (i.e. if the null hypothesis is true). It measures how well the observed (actual) distribution of data fits with the expected distribution under the null hypothesis (no difference between results).

It is obtained by calculating the squared difference between the observed and expected data, divided by the expected data in all possible categories, then summing them. On its own, this value is difficult to interpret and therefore it is given with a p-value. This is determined from a corresponding table.

The larger the difference between the observed and expected results, the larger the Chi-squared value and the smaller the corresponding p-value. The p-value tells you the strength of the evidence against the null hypothesis that the true difference in the population is zero, i.e. there is no real difference between the groups.

Clinical application/worked example

1. *Calculate the Chi-squared value of the following results from an influenza vaccine trial carried out during an epidemic.*

Observed data (o)				**Expected data* (e)**			
Influenza				Influenza			
	Yes	No	Total		Yes	No	Total
Vaccine	20	220	240	Vaccine	52.2	187.8	240
Placebo	80	140	220	Placebo	47.8	172.2	220
Total	100	360	460	Total	100	360	460

* i.e. if the vaccine and placebo were equally effective, we'd expect the same proportion in each of the two groups.

Outcome	Exposure	Observed (o)	Expected (e)	$(o - e)^2/e$
Influenza	Vaccine	20	52.2	19.86
Influenza	Placebo	80	47.8	21.69
No Influenza	Vaccine	220	187.8	5.52
No Influenza	Placebo	140	172.2	6.02
Total		460	460	53.09

Therefore $\chi^2 = 53.09$.

The *p*-value for this test, obtained from the table, is $p < 0.001$, i.e. there is strong evidence against the null hypothesis of no effect of the vaccine on the probability of contracting influenza.

Likelihood ratio

$$LR = \frac{Sensitivity}{(1 - Specificity)}$$

Definition of terms used

Sensitivity = $TP / (TP + FN)$
Specificity = $TN / (TN + FP)$
where:
TP = true positive
FP = false positive
TN = true negative
FN = false negative

Units

Fraction.

Explanation

The likelihood ratio uses sensitivity (refer to page 174) and specificity (refer to page 172) to measure how much more probable it is that a test result would be expected in a patient with a disease compared to the likelihood that the same test result would occur in a patient without the disease. It is the probability of a person who has the disease testing positive divided by the probability of a person without the disease testing positive.

LR >1 indicates that the test result is associated with the disease.

LR < 1 indicates that the result is associated with absence of the disease.

The equation uses fractions not percentages.

Clinical application/worked example

1. Calculate the likelihood ratio for this new screening test for abdominal aortic aneurysms.

New test outcome	Condition present (as determined by gold standard testing)	
	Present	Not present
Positive	32 (TP)	7 (FP)
Negative	5 (FN)	131 (TN)

(i) **Sensitivity = TP/(TP + FN)**

= 32/(32 + 5)

= 86%

(ii) **Specificity = TN/(TN + FP)**

= 131/(131 + 7)

= 95%

(iii) $LR = \dfrac{\textbf{Sensitivity}}{\textbf{(1 - Specificity)}}$

= 86/(100 − 95)

= 17.2

Standard error of mean

$$SEM = SD / \sqrt{(n)}$$

Definition of terms used

SEM = standard error of mean
SD = standard deviation
n = number of observations

Units

Nil.

Explanation

The standard error (SEM) of mean is an estimate of how close to the population mean your sample mean is likely to be, i.e. a measure of the precision of your sample mean as an estimate of the population mean. This is in contrast, and often confused with, the standard deviation (refer to page 189), which measures the amount of variability in the population and describes how individual observations within the sample differ from the population mean.

As the SEM depends on the standard deviation and sample size, as sample size increases, the standard error of mean will decrease. The larger the sample size, the smaller the standard error. By contrast, standard deviation will not be affected by sample size.

Clinical application/worked example

1. The low-density lipoproteins (LDL) cholesterol levels of 3293 subjects in a study have mean 189 mg/dl and standard deviation 19 mg/dl. Calculate the standard error of mean.

$$SEM = SD / \sqrt{(n)}$$
$$SEM = 19 / \sqrt{(3293)}$$
$$= 0.33$$

Standard deviation and variance

$$SD = \sqrt{variance}$$

And

$$Variance = SD^2 = \frac{\Sigma(x - \bar{x})^2}{(n - 1)}$$

Definition of terms used

SD = standard deviation
Σ = the sum of
x = individual observation
$\bar{x}$ = mean of all observations
n = number of observations in a sample

Units

Has the same units as the observations (e.g. mg).

Explanation

The standard deviation (SD) describes how spread out a set of observations are from the mean (i.e. the variability or deviation of each observation from the mean value).

It is equal to the square root of the variance (the average of the squares of the differences from the mean) in four easy steps.

(1) Calculate the mean for all the values ($\bar{x}$).
(2) For each individual observation (x), subtract the mean ($\bar{x}$) and square the results (to make all positive). This is known as the squared deviation.
(3) Add all the observations together (Σ) and divide by the total number of observations (n).
(4) Take the square root of the variance.

With the mean taken as the centre point, a range of one SD above (+) and below (−) will include 68.3% of the values, ± 2 SD will include 95.4% of the values, and ± 3 SD will include 99.7% of the values.

Standard deviation should only be used as a summary statistic when the data have a normal distribution. To rapidly estimate whether this is the case, calculate 2SD above and below the mean, to see if the values are possible for the variable in question.

NB: If you are sampling a small number of observations ($n < 30$), divide by 'n'. If you are sampling from a large number of observations ($n > 30$), divide by '$n - 1$'. This is called Bessel's correction and it corrects for bias in the estimation of the population variance.

Clinical application/worked example

1. *Calculate the standard deviation of the following measured LDL cholesterol levels of 4 healthy adults:*

185, 191, 187, 193 mg/dl

$n = 4$

mean ($\bar{x}$) = 189 mg/dl

To ease calculations, place data into a table:

	LDL x	Deviation from the mean $x - \bar{x}$	Squared deviation $(x - \bar{x})^2$
	185	−4	16
	191	2	4
	187	2	4
	193	4	16
Total	756	0	40

$$\textbf{\textit{Variance}} = \textbf{\textit{SD}}^2 = \frac{\Sigma(x - \bar{x})^2}{(n - 1)}$$

$$\textbf{\textit{SD}} = \sqrt{\frac{40}{3}}$$

$$= 3.65 \text{ mg/dl}$$

Power

Power = 1 − β

Definition of terms used

β = false negative rate

Units

Nil.

Explanation

The power of a statistical study measures the test's ability to reject the null hypothesis when it is actually false (a Type II error) – i.e. make the correct decision. Given that the probability of a Type II error occurring is referred to as the false negative rate (β), and as power increases the chances of a Type II error occurring decrease, power is therefore equal to 1 − β.

A Type II error would occur, for example, if a study concluded that two drugs produced the same effect (i.e. the null hypothesis, there is no difference between the drugs on average) when they actually produce different effects. Type II errors frequently occur due to small sample sizes.

Power is calculated between 0 and 1, where 1 is the 'ideal' power with no chances of a Type II error occurring.

Clinical application/worked example

1. Discuss factors that affect the statistical power for a study.

Factors include the following.
 (i) The sample size (n) used in the study.
 (ii) The magnitude of the effect of interest in the population.
 (iii) The statistical significance criterion used in the study, e.g $p < 0.05$.

Odds ratio

$$OR = \frac{\text{odds of disease in exposed individuals}}{\text{odds of disease in unexposed individuals}}$$

which is the same as

$$OR = \frac{(\text{n exposed} + \text{ve cases} / \text{n exposed} - \text{ve cases})}{(\text{n unexposed} + \text{ve cases} / \text{n unexposed} - \text{ve cases})}$$

or

$$OR = (a/b)/(c/d)$$

Definition of terms used

OR = odds ratio
a, b, c, d = as defined below

Units

Nil.

Explanation

The odds ratio is a measure of association between an exposure and an outcome. It represents the odds of an event (e.g. occurrence of a disease) happening in one group (i.e. exposure group), compared to the odds of it happening in the other group (i.e. unexposed group).

It can be used to calculate whether a particular exposure is a risk factor for a particular event or outcome, and furthermore can compare the magnitude of various risk factors for that outcome.

OR = 1: exposure does not affect odds of outcome.

OR >1: exposure associated with higher odds of outcome.

OR < 1: exposure associated with lower odds of outcome.

If a disease is rare, the odds ratio is approximately the same as the risk ratio, and can be interpreted in the same way.

Clinical application/worked example

1. It has been theorized that exposure to phenytoin increases your risk of developing drug-induced lupus. Calculate the odds ratio for this association.

Phenytoin	Drug-induced lupus	
	Positive	Negative
Yes	25	73
No	13	64

$$OR = \frac{((n) \text{ exposed} + \text{ve cases}/(n) \text{ exposed} - \text{ve cases})}{((n) \text{ unexposed} + \text{ve cases}/(n) \text{ unexposed} - \text{ve cases})}$$

$OR = (25/73)/(13/64) = 0.34/0.20$

$= 1.7$

Exposure to phenytoin is associated with a higher odds of drug-induced lupus.

Appendix 1: The International System of Units

The International System of Units, normally abbreviated to SI units, is the modern form of the metric system. It includes a comprehensible system of units of measurement developed around seven SI base units assumed to be mutually independent.

SI base units

Base quantity	Name	Symbol
Length	Metre	m
Mass	Kilogram	kg
Time	Second	s
Electric current	Ampere	A
Thermodynamic temperature	Kelvin	K
Amount of substance	Mole	mol
Luminous intensity	Candela	cd

SI-derived units

SI derived units are defined in terms of the seven base quantities using a system of quantity equations. Twenty-two of these are named.

Derived quantity	Name	Symbol	Expressed in terms of other SI units	Expressed in terms of other SI base units
Plane angle	Radian	rad	–	$m \cdot m^{-1} = 1$
Solid angle	Steradian	sr	–	$m^2 \cdot m^{-2} = 1$
Frequency	Hertz	Hz	–	s^{-1}
Force	Newton	N	–	$m \cdot kg \cdot s^{-2}$
Pressure	Pascal	Pa	N/m^2	$m^{-1} \cdot kg \cdot s^{-2}$
Energy	Joule	J	$N \cdot m$	$m^2 \cdot kg \cdot s^{-2}$
Power	Watt	W	J/s	$m^2 \cdot kg \cdot s^{-3}$
Electric charge	Coulomb	C	–	$s \cdot A$
Electric potential difference	Volt	V	W/A	$m^2 \cdot kg \cdot s^{-3} \cdot A^{-1}$
Electric capacitance	Farad	F	C/V	$m^{-2} \cdot kg^{-1} \cdot s^4 \cdot A^2$
Electric resistance	Ohm	Ω	V/A	$m^2 \cdot kg \cdot s^{-3} \cdot A^{-2}$
Electric conductance	Siemens	S	A/V	$m^{-2} \cdot kg^{-1} \cdot s^3 \cdot A^2$
Magnetic flux	Weber	Wb	$V \cdot s$	$m^2 \cdot kg \cdot s^{-2} \cdot A^{-1}$
Magnetic flux density	Tesla	T	Wb/m^2	$kg \cdot s^{-2} \cdot A^{-1}$
Inductance	Henry	H	Wb/A	$m^2 \cdot kg \cdot s^{-2} \cdot A^{-2}$
Celsius temperature	Degree Celsius	°C	–	K
Luminous flux	Lumen	lm	$cd \cdot sr$	$m^2 \cdot m^{-2} \cdot cd = Cd$
Illuminance	Lux	lx	lm/m^2	$m^2 \cdot m^{-4} \cdot cd = m^{-2} \cdot Cd$
Radioactivity	Becquerel	Bq	–	s^{-1}
Absorbed dose (of ionizing radiation)	Gray	Gy	J/kg	$m^2 \cdot s^{-2}$
Dose equivalent (of ionizing radiation)	Sievert	Sv	J/kg	$m^2 \cdot s^{-2}$
Catalytic activity	Katal	kat	–	$s^{-1} \cdot mol$

Appendix 2: Units of measurement

Prefix	Symbol	Multiplying factor
Pico	p	10^{-12}
Nano	n	10^{-9}
Milli	m	10^{-3}
Centi	c	10^{-2}
Deci	d	10^{-1}
Deca	da	10
Hecto	h	100
Kilo	K	1,000
Mega	M	1,000,000
Giga	G	1,000,000,000

Index

Terms from Chapter titles in the list of Contents are not included

Printed in the United States
By Bookmasters

Printed in the United States
By Bookmasters